Metabolism

Metabolism

Claude A. Villee, PhD
Andelot Professor of Biologic Chemistry
Laboratory of Human Reproduction and Reproductive Biology
Harvard Medical School
Boston, Massachusetts

CREOG

Basic Science Monograph in Obstetrics and Gynecology

Council on Resident Education in Obstetrics and Gynecology
600 Maryland Avenue, SW, Washington DC 20024

Library of Congress Cataloging in Publication Data
Villee, Claude Alvin, 1917-

Metabolism.

   (Basic science monograph in obstetrics and gynecology)
   Bibliography: p. 161
   Includes index.
   1. Metabolism   I. Title.   II. Series
QP171.V55 1984   612'.39   84-22997
ISBN 0-915473-02-X
1 2 3 4 5 / 8 7 6 5 4

**The development of this Basic Science Monograph
in Metabolism was made possible by a grant from
Parke-Davis.**

Contents

Preface

Modern medical practice is characterized by the degree to which it is based on scientific fact. Practice by intuition or anecdotal experiences, which may have been laudable at one point in medical history, is now condemned because it cannot withstand, or is not subjected to, the scrutiny of "scientific method." Therefore, the quality of a physician's practice is greatly influenced by the extent of the individual's scientific knowledge.

Medical education reflects a marked heterogeneity—in both the academic setting of medical school and the clinical orientation of residency programs. Today's rapid pace of scientific discoveries has an impact on the practice of obstetrics and gynecology. This fact dictates the continuing identification of basic science information most pertinent to the specialty.

In response to this need, the Council on Resident Education in Obstetrics and Gynecology (CREOG), under the direction of the CREOG Committee on Education and Curriculum, has developed a series of basic science monographs. These monographs are designed to review principles related to, but not necessarily clinically correlated with, direct patient care. The information in this series has been carefully selected to form a foundation for the application of basic science principles in a clinical environment. Such a background is an essential part of postgraduate education—both in residency and in continuing medical education.

Intentionally, the monographs are neither all encompassing nor exhaustively detailed; textbooks and other reference sources are available for more in-depth study. Rather, the review of basic science as reflected in this monograph series serves as a basis for discussion, amplification, and exploration of information particularly relevant to reproductive health. The content will be reviewed periodically and, based on critiques and feedback received, revised to ensure currency and applicability to the specialty.

To enhance the authoritativeness and usefulness of the monographs, specialists well versed in their respective fields were invited to serve as authors. CREOG is indebted to Claude A. Villee, PhD, for writing the text of this monograph on *Metabolism,* which in six chapters, outlined and indexed in detail, provides an overview of metabolic principles and mechanisms that are particularly relevant to obstetrics and gynecology.

1

Bioenergetics

The never-ending flow of energy within a cell, from one cell to another, and from one organism to another is the essence of life itself. Any interference with this flow of energy constitutes a threat to life. Living cells have within them complex, organized, efficient systems for transferring one type of energy into another. Energy—the capacity to do work—may take the form of heat, light, electricity, motion, or chemical energy. The chemical and enzymatic reactions of cells that provide for their growth, irritability, movement, maintenance, repair, and reproduction are collectively termed metabolism.

The metabolic activities of bacteria, plant cells, and animal cells are remarkably similar despite the marked differences in their appearances. In all cells, glucose and other simple sugars are converted by a series of intermediate compounds to carbon dioxide and water. During this conversion, a part of the energy of the glucose molecule is conserved and made available to drive other processes. The study of energy transformations in living organisms, termed bioenergetics, is concerned with three major questions: 1) How do cells obtain biologically useful energy? 2) How do they utilize it in synthesizing their own cellular constituents? and 3) How are these functions controlled so that they meet the moment-to-moment needs of the cells?

THERMODYNAMICS

In thermodynamic terms a *system* is the energy and matter within a defined region; the energy and matter in the rest of the universe are the *surroundings*. The first law of thermodynamics states that the total energy of a system and its surroundings is constant, that energy is conserved. Only changes in energy are measurable, however; the absolute energy of a system cannot be determined. When a system interacts with its surroundings, the amount of energy gained (or lost) by the system is exactly equal to the amount of energy lost (or gained) by the surroundings. The first law can be stated mathematically as

$$\Delta E = E_F - E_I = Q - W \tag{1}$$

E_I and E_F are the energy of a system at the beginning and end, respectively, of a process; and Q is the heat absorbed, and W is the work done by the system. As any given system undergoes a change from its initial state E_I, to its final state, E_F, it may absorb energy from the surroundings or deliver energy to the surroundings.

Nearly every physical and chemical event is associated with either the delivery of heat to the surroundings (i.e., an exothermic process) or the absorption of heat from the surroundings (i.e., an endothermic process). Although heat is a simple and familiar means of transferring energy in man-made machines, it is not a useful way of transferring energy in biologic systems for the simple reason that living systems are isothermal. There is no significant temperature difference between different parts of a cell or between different cells in the body. Cells cannot act as heat engines; they have no mechanism for heat to flow from a warmer to a cooler body.

The second law of thermodynamics, stated briefly as "the entropy of the universe increases," can be used to predict whether a reaction can occur spontaneously. Entropy (S) is a measure of the degree of randomness or disorder of a system. The entropy of a system increases, that is, ΔS becomes positive, as the system becomes more disordered. In almost all energy transformations, some heat is lost to the surroundings; since heat involves the random motion of molecules, such heat losses increase the entropy of the surroundings. Living organisms and their component cells are highly organized and thus have low entropy. They preserve this low entropy by increasing the entropy of their surroundings. For example, people increase the entropy of their surroundings when they eat a candy bar, convert its glucose to carbon dioxide and water, and return them to the surroundings.

The force that drives all processes is the tendency to reach the state of maximum entropy by giving up or absorbing heat from the surroundings. Thus the second law of thermodynamics may be rephrased: a process can occur spontaneously only if the sum of the entropies of the system and its surroundings increases. The entropy of a system may decrease during a spontaneous process if the entropy of the surroundings increases enough so that the sum of the two is positive: $\Delta S_{sys} + \Delta S$ surroundings > 0.

FREE ENERGY

Entropy is not a useful criterion of whether a biochemical process can proceed spontaneously, because changes in entropy are not readily measured. The changes in heat and entropy of a system are related by a third dimension of energy termed *free energy*. This thermodynamic function, denoted by the symbol G, was devised by Josiah Willard Gibbs over a century ago when he combined the first and second laws in the equation:

$$\Delta G = \Delta H - T\Delta S \qquad (2)$$

H is the enthalpy or total heat content of the system, and T is the absolute temperature. Free energy may be visualized as that component of the total energy of a system that is available to do work under isothermal conditions; it is thus the thermodynamic parameter of greatest interest in biology. As entropy (S) increases during an irreversible process, the amount of free energy (G) decreases. The change in free energy, ΔG, is equal to the change in the total heat content of the system, ΔH, minus the change in entropy multiplied by the absolute temperature, $T\Delta S$. All physical and chemical processes tend to proceed until they reach an equilibrium in which the free energy of the system is at a minimum and the entropy is at a maximum.

The change in free energy of a reaction can be used to determine whether the reaction can occur spontaneously. A reaction can occur spontaneously only if ΔG is negative. If ΔG is 0, the system is at equilibrium; no net change can occur. If ΔG is positive, the reaction cannot occur spontaneously; an input of free energy is necessary to drive the reaction.

The ΔG of a reaction is the free energy of the final state, the products, minus that of the initial state, the reactants. It is independent of both the path of the transformation and the mechanism of the reaction. The conversion of glucose to carbon dioxide and water has the same ΔG whether it occurs by combustion in a bomb calorimeter or by a long series of enzyme-catalyzed reactions in a living cell. Furthermore, the magnitude of the ΔG does not determine the rate of the reaction. The rate of the reaction depends on the energy of activation, E_a, which is not related to ΔG.

Most chemical reactions are reversible. The energy relations of the reactants and products, their relative concentrations, and their solubility are some of the factors that determine whether a reaction will occur and whether it will proceed from right to left or from left to right such as $A + B \rightleftarrows C + D$. For each reaction, the thermodynamic equilibrium constant, K_{eq}, expresses the chemical equilibrium reached by the system:

$$K_{eq} = \frac{(C) \times (D)}{(A) \times (B)} \tag{3}$$

The K_{eq} is unchanging and is determined by the tendency of the reaction components to reach a state of maximum entropy or minimum free energy for the system. Thus the equilibrium constant K_{eq} is related mathematically to the change in free energy of the components of the reaction:

$$\Delta G^0 = -RT \ln K_{eq} \tag{4}$$

R is the gas constant (1.987 calorie/mole-degree), T the absolute temperature, and $\ln K_{eq}$ the natural logarithm (base e) of the equilibrium constant. The symbol ΔG^0 represents the standard free energy change, defined as the free energy change for the reaction under standard conditions, when the reactants and products are present at concentrations of 1 M.

The change in free energy of the reaction $A + B \rightleftarrows C + D$ is given by the equation

$$\Delta G = \Delta G^0 + RT \ln \frac{(C)\ (D)}{(A)\ (B)} \tag{5}$$

The change in free energy, ΔG, is a function of the nature of the reactants (described in the ΔG^0 term) and of their concentrations (given in the logarithmic term). When the product $C \times D$ is equal to the product $A \times B$, $\dfrac{C \times D}{A \times B}$ equals 1, the logarithm of 1 equals 0 and the $RT \ln \dfrac{(C)\ (D)}{(A)\ (B)}$ term becomes 0; ΔG is equal to ΔG^0.

At equilibrium, when ΔG is 0,

$$0 = \Delta G^0 + RT \ln \frac{(C) \times (D)}{(A) \times (B)}$$

or, rearranging,

$$\Delta G^0 = -RT \ln \frac{(C) \times (D)}{(A) \times (B)} \tag{6}$$

Examination of Equation 4 reveals that when the equilibrium constant K_{eq} is large, the standard free energy change, ΔG^0, is negative. A reaction under these circumstances (i.e., an exergonic reaction) proceeds with a decrease in free energy. A reaction that occurs when the equilibrium constant is small and the free energy change is positive (i.e., an endergonic reaction) is not completed, however, unless additional energy is put into the system. When K_{eq} is 1, the change in free energy is 0 and the reaction is freely reversible. The standard free energy change, ΔG^0, provides a means of comparing the potential energy of different reactions. It is the calculated free energy change at defined standard concentrations, 1 M for all reactants and products and, unless otherwise specified, at 25 C, 1 atm pressure, and pH 7.

From Equation 4, it follows that the standard free energy change, ΔG^0, is a logarithmic function of the equilibrium constant. The standard free energy change for the sum of two reactions is the sum of the standard free energy changes of the individual reactions. This is very useful in considering biochemical systems in which a long sequence of reactions occurs: $A \rightarrow B, B \rightarrow C, C \rightarrow D$, for the ΔG^0 for $A \rightarrow D$ is the sum of the individual values for each step. In such a sequence, one or more of the reactions may have a positive value for ΔG^0, yet the whole sequence occurs if the sum of the reactions has a negative standard free energy change.

Glucose-1-phosphate and glucose-6-phosphate are interconverted in muscle and liver cells by a reaction catalyzed by the enzyme phosphoglucomutase. To measure the equilibrium constant and free energy change of this reaction, an adequate amount of the enzyme is added to a carefully measured amount of glucose-1-phosphate and the amounts of glucose-1-phosphate and glucose-6-phosphate are measured in the reaction mixture at succeeding times until no further change occurs (i.e., until equilibrium is reached). At equilibrium, there is 19 times more glucose-6-phosphate than glucose-1-phosphate, and the equilibrium constant, K_{eq}, is 19. Substituting this in the equation $\Delta G^0 = -RT \ln K_{eq} = -2.303\ RT \log_{10} K_{eq}$, $= -2.303 \times 1.98 \times 298 \times \log_{10} 19\ (1.28) = -1745$ calories/mol. There is a decline in free energy of 1,745 calories when 1 mol glucose-1-phosphate is converted to 1 mol glucose-6-phosphate at 25°C.

Comparable experiments show that the K_{eq} for the isomerization of dihydroxyacetone phosphate to glyceraldehyde-3-phosphate, a reaction that occurs in glycolysis, is 0.0475; ΔG^0 is $-2.303 \times 1.987 \times 298 \times \log_{10} 0.0475$, or $+1,800$ calories/mol. This endergonic reaction requires the input of energy under standard conditions with reactant and product at concentrations of 1M. At lower concentrations, however, such as 2×10^{-4}M for the reactant (i.e., dihydroxyacetone phosphate) and 2×10^{-6}M for the product (i.e., glyceraldehyde-3-phosphate), the $\Delta G = \Delta G^0 + RT \ln [\text{product}/\text{reactant}]$. Substituting these values in the equation gives

$$\Delta G - +1,800 \text{ calories/mol} \mid 1.98 \times 298 \times 2.303 \log_{10} \frac{3 \times 10^{-6}\text{M}}{2 \times 10^{-4}\text{M}}$$

or

$$\Delta G = +1,800 \text{ calories/mol} - 2,500 \text{ calories/mol, or} -700 \text{ calories/mol}$$

This negative value for ΔG implies that the isomerization of dihydroxyacetone phosphate to glyceraldehyde-3-phosphate can occur spontaneously under these conditions. This also shows that ΔG can be larger, smaller, or the same as ΔG^0, depending on the concentration of the reactants and products. Whether a reaction can occur spontaneously is determined by the ΔG, not by the ΔG^0.

Coupled Reaction Systems

Metabolic pathways are made up of sequences of reactions, each catalyzed by its specific enzyme. Two or more reactions are said to be "coupled" if a product of one reaction is a reactant in the other. The inside of a cell can be viewed as a factory with many different assembly (and disassembly) lines that operate simultaneously. Each assembly line involves a number of enzymes; one enzyme converts molecule A into molecule B, for example, and then passes it along to the next enzyme, which converts molecule B into molecule C.

Consider the following sequence of reactions:

$A \rightleftarrows B$	$\Delta G^0 = -5,000$ calories/mol
$B \rightleftarrows C$	$\Delta G^0 = +2,000$ calories/mol
$C \rightleftarrows D$	$\Delta G^0 = -3,000$ calories/mol
Sum: $A \rightleftarrows D$	$\Delta G^0 = -6,000$ calories/mol

As mentioned earlier, the overall free energy change for a series of reactions equals the algebraic sum of the free energy changes of the individual steps. In this series, reactant A is converted to product D, because the sum of the ΔG^0s is less than 0, even though one of the steps has a positive ΔG^0. Under standard conditions, B is not converted to C, because the ΔG^0 is positive. The conversion of C to D is thermodynamically feasible, however, as is the conversion of A to B. Because the free energy changes of the sequence of reactions are additive, the conversion of A to D has a ΔG^0 of $-6,000$ calories/mol and can occur under standard conditions. Even though reaction $B \rightleftarrows C$ would go spontaneously from right to left, the preceding conversion of A to B *increases* the concentration of B, while the following conversion of C to D *decreases* the concentration of C. Thus, the conversion of A to B "pushes" reaction $B \rightleftarrows C$ to the right, while the conversion of C to D "pulls" it to the right. The two exergonic reactions combine to drive the endergonic reaction, since the overall free energy change of the sequence of reactions is less than 0.

In any coupled system in which the sum of the free energy changes of the reaction is less than 0, reactants are converted to products, and material flows from left to right. The number of reactions in the sequence, the number of starting materials, and the number of end products in any given reaction are all unimportant. Only one common intermediate between two consecutive reactions is required in a coupled system. The nature of the common intermediate is also unimportant; it can be as simple as an electron or proton, or as complex as a polypeptide or polynucleotide.

Adenosine Triphosphate: The Primary "Energy Currency" of the Cell

All the phenomena of life (e.g., growth, movement, irritability, reproduction) require the expenditure of energy by the cell and a corresponding continual input of free energy. Cells use free energy for the synthesis of substances from simpler precursors, for the active transport of molecules and ions across membranes, and for the performance of mechanical work, such as the contraction of muscle and the beating of cilia. Free energy is used to maintain the organism in a state that is far from equilibrium, with a minimum of entropy and a maximum of free energy. Plants derive free energy from the light energy trapped in photosynthesis; animals and other heterotrophs, such as fungi, derive it from the oxidation of foodstuffs. The free energy thus obtained is transformed into a special carrier of free energy, adenosine triphosphate (ATP).

The biologic problem of combining markedly exergonic reactions, such as the oxidation of glucose, with tremendously endergonic reactions, such as the synthesis of a peptide from amino acids, was solved by modifying both reactions so that they have a common intermediate, a compound produced by one and used in the other—ATP. The exergonic cleavage of the nucleoside triphosphates converts an otherwise endergonic synthesis of peptides into an overall exergonic reaction. In the oxidation of glucose, the resynthesis of the ATP and guanosine triphosphate (GTP) used in peptide synthesis permits the synthesis of peptides to be "driven" by the oxidation of glucose. A markedly exergonic process, the oxidation of glucose, is modified so that nucleoside diphosphates and monophosphates are phosphorylated to form nucleoside triphosphates. This decreases the liberation of free energy that would otherwise accompany the oxidation of glucose. The nucleoside triphosphates are then used in endergonic processes and are cleaved in these reactions to diphosphates or monophosphates. Although the overall effect is that of a direct transfer of energy, the biochemical mechanism involved is a coupling of exergonic and endergonic reactions in which the nucleoside triphosphates serve as "energy carriers."

ATP is an energy-rich molecule because its triphosphate moiety contains two phosphoanhydride bonds. A large amount of free energy is liberated when ATP is hydrolyzed to adenosine diphosphate (ADP) and inorganic phosphate (P_i) or to adenosine monophosphate (AMP) and pyrophosphate (PP_i). In contrast, the hydrolysis of the phosphate of AMP to form free adenosine yields much less free energy. This reaction is the hydrolysis of a phosphate ester, the splitting of a bond between an alcohol group in adenosine and the acid group of phosphoric acid. The hydrolysis of ATP or ADP represents the cleavage of an oxygen bridge between two phosphorus atoms, the cleavage of a pyrophosphate bond, which is a reaction with a high standard free energy change. For this reason, such bonds and the compounds that contain them have been termed *energy-rich* or *high-energy* bonds.

Because the free energy of hydrolysis is not localized in the covalent bond joining the phosphorus atom to the oxygen atom, the term *energy-rich phosphate bond* is actually a misnomer. Despite this, it is a very useful term, deeply ingrained in biochemical thought by long usage. The term simply implies that the bond or compound has a large standard free energy of hydrolysis, although the free energy change is the result of changes in the chemical potential of all components of the system, including water and the hydrogen ion. Bonds are typically designated with a $\sim$ symbol if their cleavage by hydrolysis produces a large negative standard free energy change. ATP may be written $A\text{-}P\sim P\sim P$, because the final two bonds are energy-rich anhydrides whereas the bond between adenosine and the first phosphorus is an ordinary ester bond.

Some biosynthetic reactions are driven by other nucleoside triphosphates, such as GTP, uridine triphosphate (UTP), and cytidine triphosphate (CTP). The corresponding nucleoside diphosphates are GDP, UDP, and CDP. Specific enzymes catalyze the transfer of the terminal phosphate group from one nucleotide to another, for example,

$$ATP + UDP \rightleftarrows ADP + UTP$$

The features of the two terminal phosphate bonds of ATP that determine the high standard free energy of hydrolysis are not completely understood. ATP has a strong tendency to transfer its terminal phosphate group to water (i.e., ATP has a high phosphate group transfer potential). In contrast, simple phosphate esters, such as glucose-6-phosphate or glycerol phosphate, have lesser phosphate group transfer potentials and are associated with much smaller standard free energy changes.

Since the magnitude of the ΔG^0 depends on the difference in the free energies of the products and reactants, two features of the system are of importance in determining the phosphate group transfer potential: electrostatic repulsion and resonance stabilization. At pH 7, the triphosphate group of ATP bears four negative charges that repel each other strongly because of their proximity. The electrostatic repulsion between these negatively charged groups is decreased when ATP is hydrolyzed. ADP and inorganic phosphate have a greater number of resonance forms of similar energy than does ATP, and this resonance stabilization of the products contributes to the high group transfer potential of ATP.

There are other compounds with a high phosphate group transfer potential. Indeed, phosphoenol pyruvate, acetyl phosphate, and creatine phosphate have higher group transfer potentials than does ATP. Thus phosphoenolpyruvate can transfer its phosphoryl group to ADP to form ATP; this is one of the reactions by which ATP is generated in glycolysis. It appears to be biologically significant that the group transfer potential of ATP falls between those of other phosphorylated molecules; this permits ATP to function efficiently as a carrier of phosphoryl groups.

Electron Carriers

All living cells obtain free energy by enzymatic reactions in which electrons flow from one energy level to another. For humans and other aerobic organisms, oxygen is the ultimate electron acceptor. Electrons are removed from a molecule of some foodstuff, such as glucose or a fatty acid, and transferred, not directly to oxygen, but to a primary acceptor, either a pyridine nucleotide or a flavin nucleotide. The electrons are passed in turn from the reduced forms of the primary acceptors to oxygen via the electron transport system located on the inner membranes of the mitochondria. Oxygen then reacts with electrons and with hydrogen ions (protons) to form a molecule of water.

Energy-rich phosphate bonds, $\sim P$, are formed during the flow of electrons through the primary acceptors and the electron transport system. This flow of electrons has been termed the "electron cascade" and compared to a series of waterfalls, each driving a "waterwheel," an enzymatic reaction in which the energy of the electron is captured in a biologically useful, energy-rich form, such as ATP. The passage of electrons in the electron transport system is a series of oxidation and reduction reactions termed biologic oxidation. When the energy of this flow of electrons is captured in the form of $\sim P$, the process is called oxidative phosphorylation. In most biologic systems, two electrons and two protons (i.e., two hydrogen atoms) are removed together and the process termed *dehydrogenation*. Electrons removed from substrate molecules and transferred to primary acceptors, the pyridine nucleotides, may also be used directly in biosyntheses.

Two of the primary electron acceptors of the cell are the pyridine nucleotides nicotinamide adenine dinucleotide (NAD) and nicotinamide adenine dinucleotide phosphate (NADP). The reactive part of both these pyridine nucleotides is the vitamin nicotinamide. The nicotinamide ring accepts one proton and two electrons (which is equivalent to a hydride ion) from a molecule undergoing dehydrogenation, such as lactic acid, and becomes reduced NAD (i.e., NADH), releasing one proton. In comparable reactions NADP is reduced to NADPH. The pyridine nucleotide effective in the lactic dehydrogenase system is loosely bound and readily removed. Such loosely bound cofactors are termed *coenzymes*.

NAD and NADP serve as primary electron and hydrogen acceptors in dehydrogenation reactions involving substrates with the H-C-OH configuration, such as the dehydrogenation of lactic or malic acid. The two pyridine nucleotides differ in that the 2'-hydroxyl group of the adenosine moiety of NADP is esterified with phosphate. Most dehydrogenases specifically require either NAD or NADP as the electron and proton acceptor and do not react with the other; less specific enzymes react with either one, although they usually react more rapidly with one than with the other. NADPH is used primarily in reductive biosyntheses; its proton and electrons are transferred to a substrate molecule, which is then reduced. In contrast, NADH is used primarily for the generation of ATP; its electrons are transferred by the electron transport system to oxygen.

Other primary acceptors are the flavin nucleotides, flavin adenine dinucleotide (FAD) and flavin mononucleotide (FMN). Both serve in reactions involving the $-CH_2-CH_2-$ configuration, as in the dehydrogenation of succinic acid. The reactive part of the flavin nucleotides is the isoalloxazine ring of the vitamin riboflavin. Like NAD, FAD accepts two electrons; unlike NAD, it accepts both protons. The FAD of succinic dehydrogenase is bound very tightly to the protein part of the enzyme and cannot be removed easily. Such tightly bound cofactors are termed *prosthetic groups* of the enzyme.

In the absence of catalysts, the reduced pyridine nucleotides and flavin nucleotides react only very slowly or not at all with oxygen. Similarly, ATP is hydrolyzed only very slowly in the absence of a catalyst. These molecules are kinetically quite stable. Their stability is essential for their biologic function, because it enables the enzymes to control the flow of free energy and of reductive power.

The electrons of the reduced pyridine nucleotides, NADH and NADPH, must be passed through the intermediate acceptors of the electron transport system before they can react with oxygen. Although the flavin primary acceptors usually pass their electrons to the electron transport system, some flavoprotein enzymes can react directly with oxygen. When this occurs, hydrogen peroxide is produced and no $\sim$P is formed. An enzyme that mediates the removal of electrons from a substrate to a primary or intermediate acceptor is termed a dehydrogenase (e.g., lactic dehydrogenase, malic dehydrogenase, or succinic dehydrogenase); one that can mediate the transfer of electrons directly to oxygen is termed an oxidase.

Another important carrier of specific groups is coenzyme A (CoA), which contains another vitamin, pantothenic acid. CoA transfers acyl groups to specific acceptors. It is the coenzyme of acetylation, hence its name. The reactive site, to which acyl groups are linked by a thioester bond, is the terminal sulfhydryl group. The ΔG^0 for the hydrolysis of acetyl CoA is large and negative, $-7,500$ calories/mol.

$$\text{Acetyl CoA} + H_2O \rightleftarrows \text{Acetate} + \text{CoA}$$

Thus acetyl CoA has a high acetyl group transfer potential. CoA is a carrier of acetyl or acyl groups, just as ATP is a carrier of activated phosphoryl groups.

Water-Soluble Vitamins

Vitamins are relatively simple organic compounds that all plants and animals require to carry out specific metabolic functions. Although they differ widely in their structure, vitamins have in common the fact that they cannot be synthesized in adequate amounts and, hence, must be present in the diet. Some organisms can synthesize some vitamins, however. Thus what is a "vitamin" for one animal (or plant) is not necessarily one for another. For example, only guinea pigs, monkeys, and humans require ascorbic acid (vitamin C) in their diets; other animals can synthesize it from glucose. The mold *Neurospora* requires biotin. Most green plants, as well as animals, require cobalamin (vitamin B_{12}).

Two major groups of vitamins can be distinguished: those that are fat-soluble (i.e., A, D, E, and K) and those that are water-soluble (i.e., C and the B complex). The lack of any one of these vitamins produces a deficiency disease with characteristic symptoms. For example, the lack of ascorbic acid produces scurvy; the lack of thiamine, beri–beri; the lack of niacin, pellagra; and the lack of vitamin D, rickets. The vitamins with known roles in metabolism—niacin, thiamine, riboflavin, pyridoxine, pantothenic acid, biotin, folic acid, and cobalamin—have been found to be constituent parts of one or more coenzymes.

Thiamine pyrophosphate is the coenzyme for the oxidative decarboxylation of α-keto acids, such as pyruvate and α-ketoglutarate. It is also the coenzyme for transketolase. Riboflavin, as riboflavin monophosphate and FAD, is required for electron transport in the mitochondria and for certain oxidations in the endoplasmic reticulum. Because riboflavin is present in most foods and is synthesized by the intestinal bacteria, deficiencies of riboflavin are quite rare. Pyridoxine, as pyridoxal phosphate, is the coenzyme for many reactions involving amino acids (e.g., transamination, decarboxylation to amines) and for glycogen synthetase. Biotin is a coenzyme for the reactions in which carbon dioxide is added to an organic molecule, such as the conversion of pyruvate to oxaloacetate and the carboxylation of acetyl CoA to form malonyl CoA (the first step in the biosynthesis of fatty acids). Biotin is widely distributed in foods; only individuals who eat raw eggs in large quantities are likely to become deficient in biotin, since egg white contains a protein, avidin, that forms a tight complex with biotin and prevents its functioning.

Niacin is part of the coenzymes NAD and NADP, which serve as hydrogen acceptors or donors for many dehydrogenases. The vitamin folic acid appears in tetrahydrofolic acid, a coenzyme for many reactions involving one-carbon transfers, and in biopterin, the coenzyme for the conversion of phenylalanine to tyrosine. Cobalamin (vitamin B_{12}) serves as a coenzyme in certain reactions involving transfers of one-carbon compounds, such as methyl groups. Cobalamin is synthesized by bacteria, but not by higher plants or animals. Thus cobalamin is a "vitamin" for green plants, as well as for animals. Ascorbic acid is known to play a role in the hydroxylation of proline during collagen formation, but the overall function of this vitamin is still unknown.

Useful Energy from the Oxidation of Foodstuffs

Sir Hans Krebs defined three stages in the generation of energy from foodstuffs. In the first, large molecules taken in as food are cleaved into smaller units. Proteins are hydrolyzed to their constituent amino acids; polysaccharides, such as starch and glycogen, are hydrolyzed to glucose and other simple sugars; and fats are hydrolyzed to fatty acids and glycerol. No useful energy is generated at this stage, however. In the second stage, these smaller molecules are metabolized to a few simple units, such as acetyl CoA, that play a central role in metabolism. Glucose, glycerol, fatty acids, and several amino acids are converted to the acetyl unit of acetyl CoA. (A small amount of ATP is generated in certain of these metabolic pathways.) The third stage includes the citric acid cycle and oxidative phosphorylation, the final common pathways for the oxidation of foodstuffs, and the stage in which most of the ATP is generated.

The many metabolic processes that occur in the cells of humans and other organisms must be tightly regulated, yet the metabolic controls must be flexible enough to respond appropriately to changes in the internal and external environment. Metabolic regulation may be achieved by altering the catalytic activity of an enzyme in several ways. One active site on an enzyme molecule can affect the catalytic activity of another active site on the same molecule. The activity of allosteric enzymes can also be altered by regulatory molecules that are bound to sites on the enzyme other than the catalytic sites. The first reaction in a biosynthetic pathway can be inhibited allosterically by the final product of the pathway, a process known as feedback inhibition. Modification of the covalent structure of the enzyme, such as the phosphorylation of the hydroxyl group of a serine in the peptide chain, can also affect an enzyme's activity.

In the cells of humans and other eukaryotic organisms, metabolic regulation is enhanced by intracellular compartmentalization. For example, fatty acids are oxidized within the mitochondria, whereas they are synthesized in the cytosol, the soluble, nonparticulate part of the cytoplasm. This segregation of the opposing reactions in different intracellular compartments permits their separate regulation.

Energy Charge

The relative concentrations of ATP, ADP, and AMP reflect the state of energy-rich phosphates in the cell. Many metabolic reactions are controlled, at least in part, by this energy charge. The total $\sim P$ stored in the ATP–ADP–AMP system is proportional to the mole fraction of ATP plus one-half the mole fraction of ADP (ATP has two phosphoanhydride bonds, but ADP has only one):

$$\text{Energy charge} = \frac{(\text{ATP}) + \frac{1}{2}(\text{ADP})}{(\text{ATP}) + (\text{ADP}) + (\text{AMP})} \tag{7}$$

The energy charge, as defined in this equation, may have values ranging from 1 (all ATP) to 0 (all AMP). Studies by Daniel Atkinson have shown that ATP-generating pathways are inhibited by a high energy charge, whereas ATP-utilizing pathways are stimulated by a high energy charge (Fig. 1–1). When the reaction

Fig. 1–1. *Changes in the rates of ATP-generating and ATP-utilizing reactions as a function of energy charge.*

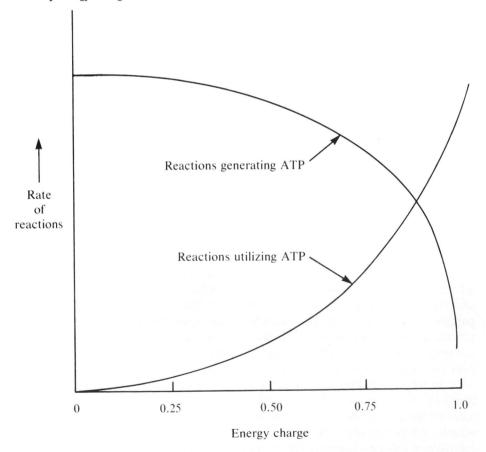

rates of such pathways are plotted against energy charge, the curves are steepest near an energy charge of 0.9, where they typically intersect. The controls of these pathways are designed to maintain the energy charge within rather narrow limits, usually between 0.8 and 0.95, by mechanisms that are analogous to the buffering mechanisms that maintain the pH of the cell within a narrow range of values.

2

Enzymes

A few of the chemical reactions that occur in biologic systems proceed without the intervention of a catalyst, but the vast majority of biochemical reactions take place only in the presence of the specific protein catalysts called enzymes. Each kind of cell in the body is characterized by a specific spectrum of enzyme activities. Some enzymes are present in essentially all the cells of the body; others are found only in one or in a very few cell types. All enzymes are proteins; some have, in addition, other nonprotein groups as integral parts of the catalytic molecule. Enzymes have enormous catalytic power; an enzyme can increase the rate of a reaction as much as 10^6 to 10^9 times over its rate in the absence of the enzyme. Carbonic anhydrase, which catalyzes the hydration of carbon dioxide to carbonic acid, H_2CO_3, increases the rate of the reaction 10^7-fold. The enzyme does not shift the equilibrium position of the reaction, but simply increases the rate at which this equilibrium position is achieved.

Enzymes are characterized by their specificity, both in the reaction that is catalyzed and in the reactants, the substrates, that participate in the reaction. Some enzymes are specific for a single type of reaction with a single type of substrate. Other enzymes catalyze a single type of reaction with a variety of substrates, and a few others are even less specific and catalyze more than one type of reaction.

All proteolytic enzymes cleave peptide bonds in a polypeptide chain, but they recognize different R groups (amino acid side chains). Trypsin, chymotrypsin, thrombin, and elastase are all serine proteases and are similar structurally; 40% of the amino acid sequences of trypsin, chymotrypsin, and elastase are identical. Their proteolytic activities are quite different, however. Trypsin cleaves a peptide bond only on the carboxyl side of lysine or arginine. Chymotrypsin cleaves the bond on the carboxyl side of aromatic amino acids, such as tryptophan, phenylalanine, and tyrosine, and at hydrophobic residues, such as methionine. Elastase cleaves peptide bonds next to amino acids with small, uncharged side groups. Thrombin recognizes and cleaves only the sequence arginine–glycine on the carboxyl side of arginine.

Some enzymes contain two or more polypeptide chains or subunits. Isozymes are groups of enzymes with similar catalytic functions and similar, but not identical, subunits. The subunits appear to be the products of different genes. The enzyme lactate dehydrogenase (LDH), for example, is made of two such subunits that combine to form a tetramer, the active enzyme. The two subunits, M and H, can combine to form five kinds of tetramers, MMMM, MMMH, MMHH, MHHH, and HHHH. The five isozymes can be separated and identified by electrophoresis. Damage to heart, muscle, or liver increases the level of LDH in the blood. The injured tissue can be identified by a comparative analysis of the isozyme pattern, since muscle LDH is predominantly of the M subunit and heart LDH is predominantly of the H subunit.

REGULATION OF ENZYMES

A cell is not simply a bag of enzymes. Individual enzymes have unique locations within the various organelles of the cell, the mitochondria, endoplasmic reticulum, nucleus, and cytosol. This localization or compartmentalization of enzymes is one means of regulating the activity of specific enzymes.

The activities of enzymes are regulated by a variety of genetic, hormonal, and feedback controls. Some enzymes are synthesized as inactive precursors that are subsequently activated at some physiologically appropriate time and place. Trypsinogen, synthesized in the acinar cells of the pancreas, is activated when enzymes in the small intestine cleave specific peptide bonds in its peptide chain to yield the active enzyme, trypsin. The sequence of enzymatic reactions in the clotting of blood provide several examples of this type of control.

Chymotrypsinogen, synthesized in the endoplasmic reticulum of the pancreatic acinar cells, is assembled in the Golgi apparatus into zymogen granules that are surrounded by a membrane. The chymotrypsinogen molecule is a peptide chain of some 245 amino acids, and it contains five disulfide bonds. Proteolytic enzymes in the gut convert this into chymotrypsin. This sort of system has an obvious advantage; these proteolytic enzymes are transported in their inactive precursor form, and only after they arrive at their place of operation in the lumen of the gut are they converted into active enzymes. When this system malfunctions, the pancreatic enzymes are converted into active enzymes while still in the pancreas, the pancreas begins to digest itself, and pancreatitis results.

The activity of an enzyme may also be controlled by the covalent insertion of a small group on one of the amino acids of the enzyme. Several enzymes, such as those that synthesize and degrade glycogen, are regulated by the attaching of a phosphoryl group to a specific serine residue in the enzyme. The insertion and removal of the phosphoryl groups are, in turn, catalyzed by specific enzymes. Under genetic control, the amount of a specific enzyme may be increased ("induced") by its substrate, or the activity may be decreased ("repressed") by its product. Enzyme activity may also be controlled directly by a variety of coenzymes, hormones, and other regulators.

In many instances, the final product of a metabolic pathway inhibits the enzyme located at the branch point where the metabolic pathway begins. For example, isoleucine, the end product, inhibits threonine deaminase, the branch point enzyme, which catalyzes the "committed step," the first of five enzymatic steps in the pathway toward the synthesis of isoleucine. When the concentration of isoleucine reaches a high level, threonine deaminase is inhibited; when the resulting decrease in the concentration of isoleucine reaches a certain point, threonine deaminase is again activated and the synthesis of isoleucine resumed. In many enzyme systems the immediate precursor of the reaction may activate the enzyme and the immediate product may inhibit it.

Enzyme activity may also be controlled by the polymerization of inactive subunits to produce an active polymer and the subsequent depolymerization of the polymer to its inactive subunits. Isocitrate has this effect on acetyl coenzyme A carboxylase, an enzyme involved in fatty acid synthesis. Enzymatic control may be achieved by energy linkage to the production of adenosine triphosphate (ATP), guanosine triphosphate (GTP), or other nucleoside triphosphates. A number of enzymes are subject to control by specific hormones. For example, adenyl cyclase, which produces 3',5'-cyclic adenosine monophosphate, is regulated by a number of peptide hormones in different tissues.

In many enzymatic reactions, not only is the substrate changed into the product, but also the energy of the reactants is converted to a different form with a high degree of efficiency. In photosynthesis, light energy is converted into chemical bond energy. In muscle, the chemical bond energy in ATP is converted into mechanical energy; in cells with sodium pumps, enzymes cleave ATP to bring about the transfer of molecules and ions across a membrane against chemical and electrical gradients.

The region of an enzyme that interacts specifically with its substrate is termed the *active site*. This is a relatively small part of the enzyme, typically some sort of cleft or crevice into which the specific substrate just fits. It may be formed by the folding of the polypeptide chain in a way that brings into proximity amino acids that are far apart in the peptide chain. Thus the three-dimensional active site of chymotrypsin is formed by a folding of the amino acid chain that brings histidine number 57 close to serine number 195. The amino acids at the enzyme's active site can bind the substrate and then attack specific susceptible bonds of the substrate. In some enzymes, the substrate changes the shape of the active site, thereby inducing enzymatic activity. This dynamic process is termed *induced fit*. The conformational changes in the enzyme may be accompanied by changes in the shape of the substrate as well. Substrates are bound to enzymes by relatively weak forces, such as ionic and hydrophobic bonds.

To be converted into product, the substrate molecules must have enough energy to enter a transition state in which bonds are likely to be made or broken. The energy required to bring molecules into the transition state is termed the free energy of activation, $\Delta G^{0\ddagger}$ or E_0. Reaction rates can be increased by raising the temperature or by decreasing the free energy of activation. Because the cells of the body are isothermal, the only way to increase the reaction rate in vivo is to decrease the free energy of activation. Catalysts in general and enzymes in particular combine transiently with the substrate to reduce the free energy of activation to a level below that of the uncatalyzed reaction. Enzymes do not alter the equilibrium of a chemical reaction; they simply decrease the time required for the system to reach equilibrium.

ENZYME KINETICS

It is assumed that substrates interact with enzymes in a way that does not permanently alter the enzymes, yet greatly facilitates the interaction of substrates. First, the substrates bind to the surface of the enzyme, forming an enzyme–substrate complex. The chemical reaction between substrates occurs while they are bound to the active site of the enzyme, yielding the reaction products that subsequently dissociate from the enzyme surface. Thus the course of a typical enzyme-catalyzed reaction can be described as

Substrate 1 + Substrate 2 + Enzyme ⇄ Complex ⇄ Product 1 + Product 2 + Enzyme

The detailed kinetic analysis of even such a relatively simple reaction is extremely complex, involving equations with hundreds of terms. The principles involved can be readily grasped by considering the simpler situation, the enzymatic conversion of a single substrate into a single product.

Irreversible Single Substrate Reaction

Let us assume that enzyme E combines reversibly with substrate S, thereby catalyzing its conversion to product P. Let us assume further that the reverse reaction, the conversion of P to S, is so slow that it can be neglected. How does the rate of formation of P vary with changes in the concentration of S? The situation can be described as follows:

$$E + S \underset{k2}{\overset{k1}{\rightleftharpoons}} ES \xrightarrow{k3} E + P$$

The rate constants, $k1$, $k2$, and $k3$, describe the velocities of the individual reactions. For example, the rate of formation of the enzyme–substrate complex is proportional to the product of the concentrations of the reactants, E and S. The rate of complex formation is $k1$ [E] [S], while the rate of product formation (the catalytic rate) depends only on the concentration of the enzyme–substrate complex and the relevant rate constant: $k3$ [ES]. The initial substrate is regenerated from the enzyme–substrate complex at the rate $k2$ [ES].

The analysis begins with the steady state assumption, first made by Briggs and Haldane in 1925. They assumed that, beginning a very short time after mixing substrate and enzyme, the concentration of enzyme–substrate complex would rise and would remain constant throughout the course of the reaction. Therefore, the rate of formation of the complex could be equated with the rate of its decomposition:

$$k1 \; [E] \; [S] = k2 \; [ES] + k3 \; [ES] = (k2 + k3) \; [ES] \tag{1}$$

The total concentration of enzyme, $[E_T]$, is the sum of concentrations of free and bound enzyme:

$$[E_T] = [E] + [ES] \tag{2}$$

The overall velocity of the reaction at any moment is simply

$$v = k3 \; [ES] \tag{3}$$

Equations 1 and 2 can be solved for [ES]:

$$[ES] = \frac{[E_T] \; [S]}{(k2 + k3)/k1 + [S]} \tag{4}$$

Substituting this value for [ES] in Equation 3,

$$v = \frac{k3 \; [E_T] \; [S]}{(k2 + k3)/k1 + [S]} \tag{5}$$

describes the desired relation between reaction velocity and the substrate concentration.

Examination of this equation reveals that when [S] is very large the denominator becomes approximately equal to [S] and

$$v = k3 \; [E_T] = V_{max}$$

In other words, when [S] is so large that all the enzyme molecules have substrate bound to them, $[ES] = [E_T]$, the maximal possible velocity of the reaction, V_{max}, is obtained.

$$v = \frac{V_{max} \; [S]}{(k2 + k3)/k1 + [S]} \tag{6}$$

When the concentration of substrate is such that the observed velocity is exactly half the maximum velocity,

$$v = \frac{V_{max}}{2} = \frac{V_{max} \; [S]}{(k2 + k3)/k1 + [S]}$$

it follows that

$$[S] = \frac{k2 + k3}{k1} = K_m$$

K_m, the Michaelis–Menten constant, is defined as the concentration of substrate that results in half maximal velocity. Having defined V_{max} and K_m mathematically, we can rewrite Equation 5 as

$$v = \frac{V_{max}\,[S]}{K_m + [S]} \tag{7}$$

Equation 7, termed the Michaelis–Menten equation, relating velocity v, and substrate concentration, [S], is that of a rectangular hyperbola with V_{max} as the asymptote (Fig. 2–1).

At low concentrations of substrate, when [S] is much less than K_m, Equation 7 approaches $v = V_{max}\,[S]/K_m$ (i.e., the rate is directly proportional to [S]). At high concentrations of substrate, when [S] is much greater than K_m, Equation 7 approaches $v = V_{max}$ (i.e., the rate is maximal and independent of substrate concentration, [S].

Thus the catalytic properties of a simple enzyme can be summarized by two constants, the V_{max} and the K_m (Equation 7). Each of these mathematical constants can be given a fairly precise physical meaning. The V_{max} of an enzyme is a reflection of the rapidity with which substrate molecules, once bound on the enzyme surface, are converted to products. This property of an enzyme, termed its *turnover number,* is defined as the number of molecules of substrate that can be converted to products

Fig. 2–1. K_m, *the Michaelis-Menton constant, is the concentration of substrate that results in half maximal velocity* $(V_{max/2})$ *of the enzyme reaction.*

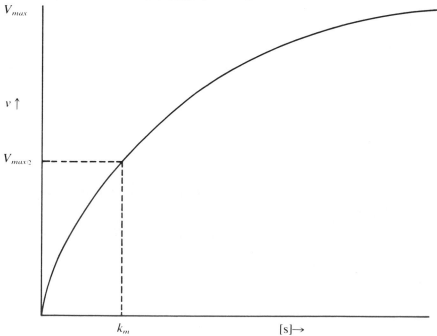

in 1 minute by one molecule of enzyme when it is saturated with substrate. Enzymes differ greatly in their turnover numbers, with values ranging from less than 1,000 to more than 10,000,000/min.

The K_m reflects a quite different property—the degree of affinity an enzyme has for its substrate. It can be defined as it was earlier, as the concentration of substrate (mol/liter) at which half of the active sites of the enzyme are filled and the velocity of the reaction is half maximal. A low K_m indicates that a relatively low concentration of substrate is needed to achieve maximal velocity. K_m is also a measure of binding affinity, a measure of the strength of the binding of enzyme to substrate to form the enzyme–substrate complex. A low K_m indicates tight binding of substrate by the enzyme. The true affinity of an enzyme for its substrate is given by the substrate dissociation constant:

$$K_s = \frac{k2}{k1}$$

This differs from the K_m only in the absence of the term $k3$ in the numerator. In some instances, $k3$ is large enough relative to $k2$ to make K_m much larger than K_s; however, it is useful to regard the K_m as a rough measure of the tightness of substrate binding.

Unfortunately, it is not easy to obtain an accurate measure of the V_{max} by eye from a plot of v versus [S] as shown in Figure 2–1. If a computer is available, the V_{max} asymptote can be calculated, and hence the K_m as well. It is customary, however, to evaluate these constants by the procedure introduced in 1934 by Lineweaver and Burk. Inverting Equation 7 and separating the terms on the right side produces

$$\frac{1}{v} = \frac{K_m}{V_{max}} \cdot \frac{1}{[S]} + \frac{1}{V_{max}} \tag{8}$$

A Lineweaver–Burk plot of $1/v$ against $1/[S]$ yields a straight line whose slope is K_m/V_{max} and whose intercepts on the y and x axes are $1/V_{max}$ and $-1/K_m$, respectively (Fig. 2–2).

Such a double reciprocal plot is useful in estimating the kinetic parameters of an enzyme, although it is evident from the plot that the reaction velocity must be measured over a wide range of substrate concentrations if an accurate determination of K_m is to be obtained.

The K_m value is useful in considering which substrate is bound preferentially when several substrates are present. The substrate with the lowest K_m is bound most effectively and competes successfully for the binding sites on the enzyme. Thus glucose (K_m 0.15 mM) is more likely to be bound to hexokinase than is fructose (K_m 1.5 mM).

The K_m of an enzyme–substrate complex may vary from one tissue to another, depending on the structure of the enzyme. Liver hexokinase has a K_m for glucose of 2×10^{-2} M, but the hexokinase of the brain has a K_m for glucose of 5×10^{-5} M.

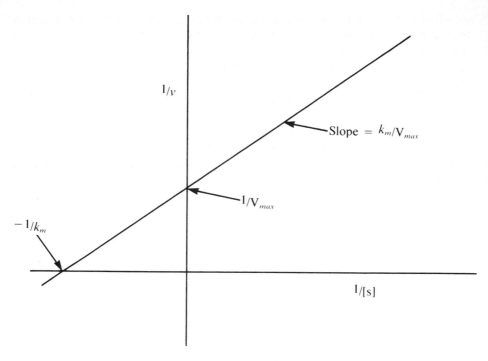

Fig. 2–2. *A Lineweaver-Burk plot of $1_{/v}$ versus $1_{/[S]}$.*

Such differences play an important role in regulating metabolism. The concentration of glucose in the blood varies from 5×10^{-3} M to 10^{-2} M, depending on the length of time since the person's last meal and the amount of exercise the person has had. The activity of the liver hexokinase is regulated by the fluctuating concentrations of glucose in the blood and tissues, since that concentration will be about the same as its K_m. In contrast, the concentration of glucose in the brain is always much higher than the K_m of the brain hexokinase, and that enzyme will always be working at maximal velocity. Since the brain uses glucose preferentially as the substrate for energy metabolism, this fact is important physiologically.

Effects of Inhibitors

Substances other than substrates may interact with an enzyme to inhibit its activity. Since reaction products are structurally similar to the substrates from which they arise, such products may act as inhibitors of the enzymes responsible for their formation (product inhibition).

COMPETITIVE INHIBITION

Inhibition is competitive when the binding of either the inhibitor or the substrate to a given enzyme molecule totally prevents the binding of the other. If an inhibitor occupies the active site of an enzyme, obviously, the substrate cannot be bound to the same site. Structural analogs of substrates are often competitive inhibitors. For example, malonic acid, HOOC-CH$_2$-COOH is a powerful competitive inhibitor of the oxidation of succinic acid, HOOC-CH$_2$-CH$_2$-COOH, by succinic dehydrogenase. Mutually exclusive binding of substrate and inhibitor can occur even when each substance binds to a different site on the enzyme. The binding of a substance to one site on a protein molecule often changes the conformation of the protein, altering the properties of the remaining binding sites.

Because of the mutually exclusive nature of the binding of substrate and inhibitor, the effectiveness of the competitive inhibitor in slowing an enzymatic reaction depends on the relative concentrations of substrate and inhibitor (I).

$$\text{E + S} \underset{k2}{\overset{k1}{\rightleftarrows}} \text{ES} \overset{k3}{\rightarrow} \text{E + P}$$

$$\text{E + I} \underset{k6}{\overset{k5}{\rightleftarrows}} \text{EI}$$

Applying the steady state assumption to the enzyme–inhibitor complex as it was applied to the enzyme–substrate complex in Equation 1 gives

$$\text{k1 [E] [S]} = \text{k2 [ES]} + \text{k3 [ES]} - (\text{k2} + \text{k3}) \text{ [ES]} \tag{9}$$

$$k5 \text{ [E] [I]} = k6 \text{ [EI]} \tag{10}$$

The total concentration of the enzyme is now given by

$$[\text{E}_\text{T}] = [\text{ES}] + [\text{EI}] + [\text{E}] \tag{11}$$

The reaction velocity at any time is as in Equation 3.

$$v = \text{k3 [ES]}$$

Rearranging Equation 10 gives

$$\frac{[\text{E}] [\text{I}]}{[\text{EI}]} = \frac{k6}{k5} = K_i \tag{12}$$

where K_i is the dissociation constant of the enzyme–inhibitor complex. Also, from Equations 9 and 10

$$[\text{ES}] = \frac{[\text{E}] [\text{S}]}{K_m} \tag{13}$$

and

$$[\text{EI}] = \frac{[\text{E}] [\text{I}]}{K_i}$$

Substituting these values into Equation 11,

$$[E_T] = \frac{[E][S]}{K_m} + \frac{[E][I]}{K_i} + [E] \tag{14}$$

$$[E] = \frac{[E_T]}{1 + [I]/K_i + [S]/K_m}$$

Inserting this value for [E] into Equation 13 for [ES]

$$[ES] = \frac{[E_T][S]}{K_m (1 + [I]/K_i) + [S]} \tag{15}$$

and finally, from Equation 3

$$v = \frac{k3 [E_T][S]}{K_m (1 + [I]/K_i) + [S]} = \frac{V_{max}[S]}{K_m (1 + [I]/K_i) + [S]} \tag{16}$$

Comparison with Equation 7 reveals that the rate equation in the presence of a competitive inhibitor is of similar form, but the K_m term is multiplied by the factor $(1 + [I]/K_i)$. The effect of this modification on a double reciprocal plot can be visualized by inverting Equation 16:

$$\frac{1}{v} = \frac{K_m (1 + [I]/K_i)}{V_{max}} \cdot \frac{1}{[S]} + \frac{1}{V_{max}} \tag{17}$$

As in the earlier illustration of velocity (see Fig. 2–2), a straight line is obtained; the slope and x intercept are however altered, (Fig. 2–3).

Thus kinetic data for reactions involving competitive inhibition yield a family of straight lines, one for each concentration of inhibitor, all of which intersect on the ordinate. If an unrecognized competitive inhibitor were present in an enzyme assay, the observed K_m would be larger than the true K_m by the factor $(1 + [I]/K_i)$. For this reason, enzymologists often refer to a calculated K_m value as an "apparent K_m."

NONCOMPETITIVE INHIBITION

In noncompetitive inhibition, the substrate and inhibitor bind independently to the enzyme, but any enzyme molecules containing bound inhibitor convert substrate to product at a reduced rate. Because the binding of substrate does not affect the binding of the inhibitor, the degree of inhibition is not influenced by the concentration of the substrate. Obviously, noncompetitive inhibitors do not interact directly with the active site of the enzyme, but influence the catalytic processes at the active site indirectly.

The derivative of the rate equation for noncompetitive inhibition is analogous to those previously given, except that a third complex, the ternary enzyme–sub-

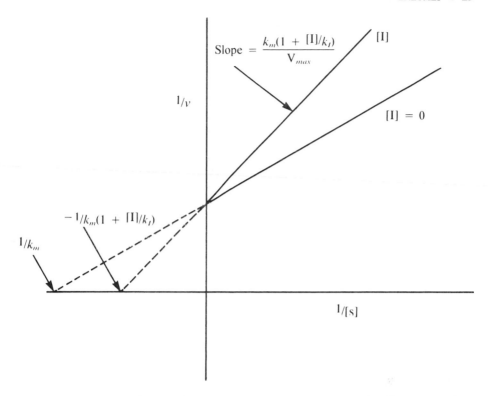

Fig. 2-3. *Lineweaver-Burk plots illustrating competitive inhibition ([I]) and uninhibited reaction ([I]=0).*

strate–inhibitor complex, must now be considered. Solving the five equations involved gives the following rate equation for noncompetitive inhibition:

$$v = \frac{V_{max} [S]}{(1 + [I]/K_i)/(K_m + [S])} \tag{18}$$

The same factor $(1 + [I]/K_i)$ appears, as was seen with competitive inhibition, but it is now the V_{max} that must be divided by this factor. The double reciprocal plot of this equation yields a family of straight lines, one for each inhibitor concentration, which intersect on the abscissa (Fig. 2-4).

$$\frac{1}{v} = \frac{K_m (1 + [I]/K_i)}{V_{max}} \cdot \frac{1}{[S]} + \frac{1}{V_{max}} (1 + [I]/K_i \tag{19}$$

The definitions of competitive and noncompetitive inhibition given here represent extreme cases. It is not unusual to encounter an intermediate mixed inhibition, in which the family of lines in a double reciprocal plot intersect at a point in the second quadrant between the ordinate and abscissa.

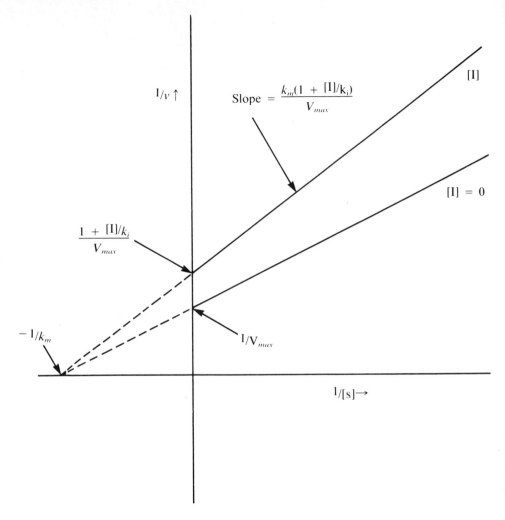

$1/v \uparrow$

$\text{Slope} = \dfrac{k_m(1 + [\text{I}]/k_i)}{V_{max}}$

[I]

[I] = 0

$\dfrac{1 + [\text{I}]/k_i}{V_{max}}$

$-1/k_m$

$1/V_{max}$

$1/[\text{s}] \rightarrow$

Fig. 2–4. *Lineweaver-Burk plot illustrating noncompetitive inhibition ([I]) in comparison with uninhibited reaction ([I]=0).*

Reversible Single Substrate Reaction

Let us consider briefly the more realistic example of a reversible single substrate reaction:

$$
\begin{array}{ccccccc}
 & k1 & & k2 & & k3 & \\
\text{E} + \text{S} & \rightleftarrows & \text{ES} & \rightleftarrows & \text{EP} & \rightleftarrows & \text{E} + \text{P} \\
 & k{-}1 & & k{-}2 & & k{-}3 &
\end{array}
$$

The situation can be analyzed by assuming steady state conditions and obtaining the following rate equation:

$$v = \frac{V_{max} \cdot K'_m \cdot [S] - V'_{max} \cdot K_m \cdot [P]}{K_m \cdot K'_m + K'_m \cdot [S] + K_m \cdot [P]} \tag{20}$$

The constants indicated with a prime are those of the reverse reaction. Both the V_{max} and the K_m are complex functions of the individual rate constants, but they have the same empirical meaning described previously. These constants are to be measured in the absence of product.

When the reaction reaches equilibrium,

$$v = 0$$

$$[S] = [S_{eq}]$$

$$[P] = [P_{eq}]$$

And Equation 20 simplifies to

$$V_{max} \cdot K'_m \cdot [S_{eq}] = V'_{max} \cdot K_m \cdot [P_{eq}]$$

or

$$\frac{V_{max}}{V'_{max}} \cdot \frac{K'_m}{K_m} - \frac{[P_{eq}]}{[S_{eq}]} = K_{eq} \tag{21}$$

This equation, called the Haldane relationship, relates the kinetic constants of an enzyme to the equilibrium constant of the reaction catalyzed. It can be seen that the equilibrium constant limits the possible values of the kinetic constants. Only three of the four terms, V_{max}, V'_{max}, K_m, and K'_m, that describe an enzyme can be considered independent variables.

By means of the Haldane relationship, the rate equation for a reversible reaction (Equation 20) can be further simplied:

$$v = \frac{V_{max} [S] - [P]/K_{eq}}{K_m (1 - [P]/K'_m) - [S]} \tag{22}$$

It can be seen that the product term in the numerator, dependent on the equilibrium constant of the reaction, limits the forward velocity of the reaction because of the occurrence of the reverse reaction; the product term in the denominator, dependent on the K'_m of the product, represents competitive inhibition of the forward reaction by the product.

Since most enzymatic reactions are in fact reversible, Equation 22 is more appropriate for their kinetic analysis than Equation 7. In order to reduce the complexity of Equation 22, enzymologists usually measure reaction velocities when the product concentration, $[P]$, is negligibly small so that Equations 22 and 7 become equivalent. Thus the initial rate of conversion of substrate to product is measured before significant amounts of product have accumulated. In the living cell, however, substantial quantities of reaction products may well be present.

3

Carbohydrates and Their Metabolism

Each cell in every organism produces a host of enzymes that catalyze the many reactions basic to life. These metabolic processes have a coherent design composed of many common motifs. Although the number of enzymatic reactions that occur in cellular metabolism is very large, the number of reaction types is relatively small. Each cell must in some way extract free energy and reducing power from the compounds in its environment. The enzymatic mechanisms used to extract free energy from compounds, such as glucose, and conserve a portion of it in the biologically useful form, $\sim P$, are very similar in the cells of animals, bacteria, and fungi. The cells of green plants carry out comparable reactions in the dark to provide energy when photosynthesis is not possible. In both animal and plant cells, many of these reactions are catalyzed by enzymes located in the mitochondria, either bound to the mitochondrial membranes or present in the fluid matrix within the mitochondria. Mitochondria have been termed the "powerhouses" of the cell.

The reactions by which cells extract energy from glucose, fatty acids, and other foodstuffs; use oxygen; and produce carbon dioxide and water are termed *cellular respiration*. There are two types of living organisms. Autotrophs, principally algae and plants, use the energy of sunlight to synthesize organic compounds, such as glucose, from carbon dioxide and water. Heterotrophs, such as animals and fungi, convert organic molecules to carbon dioxide and water, conserving some of the energy as adenosine triphosphate (ATP). Neither type could survive long without the other.

The oxidation of glucose to carbon dioxide and water in cells cannot occur in a single reaction; there are no enzymes that can catalyze the direct attack of oxygen molecules on glucose. Instead, the oxidation of glucose occurs in a lengthy sequence of reactions that can be grouped into four systems:

1. Glycolysis, the conversion of glucose to pyruvic acid with the formation of some ATP:

$$\text{Glucose} + 2 \text{ ADP} + 2 \text{ P}_i \rightarrow 2 \text{ Pyruvic acid} + 2 \text{ ATP}$$

2. Conversion of pyruvic acid to acetyl CoA (CoA) and carbon dioxide:

$$2 \text{ Pyruvic acid} \rightarrow 2 \text{ Acetyl CoA} + 2 \text{ CO}_2$$

3. Krebs tricarboxylic acid cycle, which converts acetyl CoA to carbon dioxide and removes electrons and protons:

$$2 \text{ Acetyl CoA} \rightarrow 4 \text{ CO}_2 + 8 \text{ e}^- + 8 \text{ H}^+$$

4. Electron transport system, which takes electrons removed from substrate molecules by dehydrogenases and passes them through a series of intermediate compounds so that ultimately they react with oxygen and protons to form water. As the electrons are transferred from one intermediate to the next, some of the energy is used in the synthesis of ATP from ADP and inorganic phosphate, P_i:

$$\text{ADP} + P_i + 2 \text{ e}^- + 2 \text{ H}^+ + \tfrac{1}{2}\text{O}_2 \rightarrow \text{H}_2\text{O} + \text{ATP}$$

Human beings and many other animals usually obtain more of their energy by oxidizing fatty acids than by oxidizing glucose. The fatty acids are chopped enzymatically into two-carbon compounds bound to CoA (coenzyme of acetylation). These acetyl CoA molecules enter the tricarboxylic acid cycle and are converted to carbon dioxide with the release of electrons and protons.

Energy-yielding (exergonic) reactions are coupled with energy-requiring (endergonic) reactions (see Chapter 1). In living cells, the exergonic reactions usually involve the synthesis of ATP. The central role of ATP in energy-yielding and energy-requiring reactions in biologic systems was first recognized by Fritz Lipmann and Herman Kalckar in 1941. The free energy liberated in the hydrolysis of the pyrophosphate bonds of ATP is used to drive the reactions that require an input of free energy. ATP is formed from ADP and inorganic phosphate when fuel molecules are oxidized or when light energy is trapped in photosynthesis. The basic mechanism of energy exchange in living systems is the cyclic conversion of ATP to ADP and back:

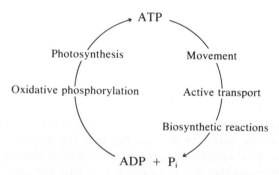

Molecules of ATP are not a storage form of energy, but they serve as immediate donors of energy in biologic systems. Cells usually contain relatively little ATP at any given moment. Because ATP molecules are typically used within a minute of their formation, the turnover of ATP molecules is very rapid. A resting 70-kg human being consumes about 50 kg ATP every 24 hours and as much as 0.5 kg/min during strenuous exercise, yet the amount present in the human body at any given moment is on the order of 0.2 g. Energy-rich phosphates are stored in muscle as creatine phosphate. The reaction

$$\text{Creatine} + \text{ATP} \rightleftarrows \text{Creatine phosphate} + \text{ADP}$$

is readily reversible. The energy-rich phosphate of creatine phosphate is readily transferred to ADP to form ATP to be used in muscle contraction.

BIOLOGIC OXIDATION AND REDUCTION

The passage of electrons from substrate molecules to oxygen in the electron transport system within the mitochondria involves a series of reactions in which the intermediates are alternately oxidized and reduced. These reactions are termed *biologic oxidation.* When the energy of this flow of electrons is used to drive the synthesis of ATP from ADP and inorganic phosphate the overall process is termed *oxidative phosphorylation.*

There is a logic and order to the array of enzymatic reactions that compose the various cycles of metabolism. The energy of ATP can be used to drive any of the many energy-requiring (endergonic) reactions of the cell. ATP is made largely in the electron transport system in the mitochondria. In principle, the energy to produce the ATP is derived from reactions in which electrons with high potential are passed through a series of compounds. Small bits of energy are extracted at each step and stored in ATP. The electrons, after giving up most of their energy to these intermediate compounds, combine with hydrogen ions (protons) and molecular oxygen to form water.

Cells need a constant supply of oxygen atoms to combine with the electrons and protons. The oxygen serves as an electron "sink," a place to put the electrons after they have given up their energy to form ATP. Without oxygen, there is no place to put the electrons, the intermediates in the electron transport system become filled with electrons, and the whole energy-producing system of the cell grinds to a halt. The cell is suffocated and dies. Some cells can survive for a brief time without oxygen by frantically moving their electrons into other compounds, such as lactic acid, but animal cells have only a very limited capacity to do this. Yeasts and certain bacteria can survive for a much longer time in the absence of oxygen.

To keep the electron transport system supplied with electrons of high potential, the dehydrogenases of the cell remove electrons from foodstuffs and transfer them to primary acceptors, such as nicotinamide adenine dinucleotide (NAD) and flavin adenine dinucleotide (FAD). In the course of evolution these have developed just the right properties for transferring electrons to the electron transport system. The cells of human beings, and the cells of animals in general, obtain most of their energy by metabolizing fats and sugars. The oxidation of fatty acids yields acetyl CoA. The metabolism of glucose and pyruvic acid also yields acetyl CoA.

The tricarboxylic acid cycle is a clever device that does indirectly what would be very difficult to do directly—split the -C-C- bond of a two-carbon compound such as acetyl CoA. It is very much easier to split a -C-C- bond that is two carbons away from a C=O group, -C–C-C=O. A similar reaction is used in splitting the -C-C- bonds in fatty acids. The two-carbon acetyl CoA condenses with the four-carbon compound, oxaloacetic acid, in an enzyme-catalyzed reaction to yield the six-carbon citric acid. The condensation product of oxaloacetic acid, citric acid can undergo a series of reactions, such as the cleavage of -C-C- bonds, and regenerate oxaloacetic acid so that it can be used over and over again. Such a system, in which the reactions eventually regenerate one of the starting materials, is termed a *catalytic cycle.* Many acetyl CoA units can be converted to carbon dioxide without exhausting the supply of oxaloacetic acid necessary for the condensation process. In the process of cleaving -C-C- bonds, electrons are removed and transferred to primary acceptors, NAD and FAD, to be passed through the electron transport system where ATP can be generated. Thus the strategy of the tricarboxylic acid cycle is to take acetyl coenzyme A units formed in the metabolism of fatty acids or sugars, combine them with oxaloacetic acid so their -C-C- bonds can be split (and obtain energy-rich electrons to pass to the primary acceptors) and regenerate the oxaloacetic acid so the catalytic cycle can continue. Marvelous!

ACTIVATION OF SUBSTRATES

In order to convert a fatty acid, such as palmitic (16 carbons long), to acetyl CoA units, the fatty acid must first be "activated," that is, a CoA unit must be added to the carboxyl group. This requires the investment of energy from ATP.

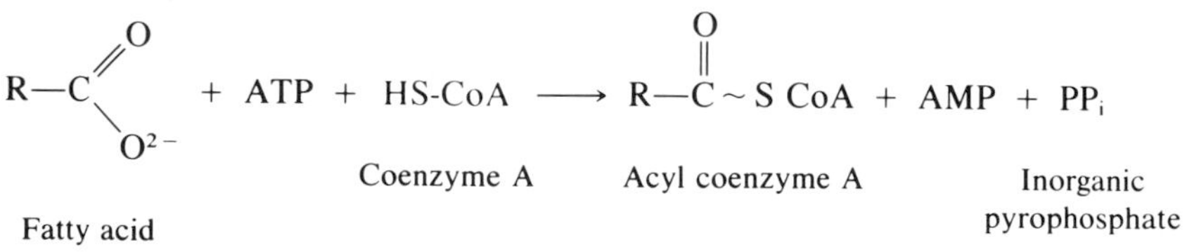

$$R—C\underset{O^{2-}}{\overset{O}{\diagup\diagdown}} + ATP + HS\text{-}CoA \longrightarrow R—\overset{O}{\overset{\|}{C}} \sim S\ CoA + AMP + PP_i$$

Fatty acid   Coenzyme A   Acyl coenzyme A   Inorganic pyrophosphate

Two energy-rich phosphates are used to drive this activation reaction. The pyrophosphate is cleaved by the enzyme pyrophosphatase to inorganic phosphate, $PP_i \rightarrow 2\ P_i$. It is this cleavage of the pyrophosphate bond that drives the union of fatty acid and CoA to the right, converting ATP to adenosine monophosphate (AMP).

Before glucose can enter metabolic pathways, it must be converted first to glucose-6-phosphate and then to fructose-1,6-diphosphate. This requires the investment of two energy-rich phosphates from ATP:

Glucose + ATP → Glucose-6-phosphate + ADP

Glucose-6-phosphate → Fructose-6-phosphate

Fructose-6-phosphate + ATP → Fructose-1,6-diphosphate + ADP

Amino acids need not be activated by reacting with ATP in order to undergo metabolism. Amino acids are oxidized by reactions in which the amino group is removed (a process termed *deamination*) and the carbon chain metabolized. The exact sequence of subsequent reactions varies somewhat with different amino acids, but a series of reactions modifies the carbon skeletons of the amino acids to produce substances that are members of the tricarboxylic acid cycle. Alanine undergoes deamination to become pyruvic acid, glutamic acid undergoes deamination to become α-ketoglutaric acid, and aspartic acid similarly yields oxaloacetic acid. These three amino acids enter the tricarboxylic acid cycle directly after they have been deaminated. Other amino acids may require in addition several enzyme-catalyzed reactions to yield a substance that is a member of the tricarboxylic acid cycle. Ultimately, the carbon chains of all amino acids are metabolized in this way.

The tricarboxylic acid cycle is the final common pathway for the metabolism of fatty acids, sugars, and amino acids to obtain carbon dioxide and water. In the reactions of the cycle, four pairs of electrons are removed and passed to the electron transport system to be used to generate ATP by oxidative phosphorylation.

DEHYDROGENATIONS, DECARBOXYLATIONS, AND "MAKE-READY" REACTIONS

The many reactions involved in cellular respiration can be assigned to one of three types:

1. Dehydrogenations are reactions in which two hydrogens (actually two electrons plus two protons) and removed from the substrate and transferred to a primary acceptor, such as NAD or FAD.
2. Decarboxylations are reactions in which a carboxyl group (-COOH) is removed as a molecule of carbon dioxide.
3. Make-ready reactions are those in which molecules undergo rearrangements so that they can subsequently undergo further dehydrogenations or decarboxylations.

Lactic acid, the acid of sour milk, is an important intermediate in cellular metabolism and can be used as an example. The molecule of lactic acid contains the structure H-C-OH, from which two hydrogens can be removed by the enzyme lactic dehydrogenase. In all dehydrogenations, the electrons removed are transferred to a primary acceptor, in this case, NAD. The product of the reaction, pyruvic acid, cannot undergo a further dehydrogenation directly, for it does not have in its molecule a suitable structure. One or more make-ready reactions are required to obtain such a structure. Therefore, pyruvic acid undergoes a decarboxylation, the removal of its carboxyl group as carbon dioxide. All of the carbon dioxide we breathe out each day is derived only by decarboxylations, by reactions such as this.

The two-carbon compound remaining reacts with a large, complex organic molecule,
CoA, and forms a substance with an H-C-OH group that can be dehydrogenated,
yielding acetyl CoA. The oxidative decarboxylation of pyruvic acid is a complex
set of reactions that require lipoic acid and thiamine pyrophosphate as cofactors,
in addition to NAD and CoA:

$$CH_3COCOOH + NAD^+ + CoA \rightarrow CH_3CO \sim SCoA + NADH + H^+ + CO_2$$

Both thiamine pyrophosphate and NAD are derivatives of B vitamins, which is
one reason that these B vitamins are so important in the body.

The oxidation of succinic acid involves the molecular structure $-CH_2-CH_2-$
and uses FAD as the primary acceptor of electrons and protons. Succinic acid is
oxidized to fumaric acid, and two of its hydrogens (two protons and two electrons)
are transferred to the flavin. Fumaric acid cannot be dehydrogenated directly, but
reacts with a molecule of water (a make-ready reaction) to yield malic acid. Malic
acid has an H-C-OH group, and malic dehydrogenase catalyzes the transfer of the
hydrogens to the primary acceptor, NAD. The product is oxaloacetic acid. This
may undergo several reactions, one of which is a decarboxylation to yield pyruvic
acid. Oxaloacetic acid may also condense with acetyl CoA to form citric acid.

GLYCOLYSIS

The sequence of reactions that convert glucose and other hexoses to pyruvic
acid with the concomitant production of ATP is exactly the same in the presence
of oxygen (termed *aerobic glycolysis*) or in the absence of oxygen (termed *anaerobic
glycolysis*). Oxygen does affect the fate of the products of glycolysis, however. In
aerobic glycolysis, pyruvic acid enters the mitochondria and is metabolized to
carbon dioxide and water by the tricarboxylic acid cycle and electron transport
system. In anaerobic glycolysis, pyruvic acid is converted to lactic acid by lactic
dehydrogenase. Some organisms, such as yeasts, have enzymes that can convert
pyruvic acid to ethanol under anaerobic conditions. If we had a similar enzyme
system we could get drunk by holding our breath and running up several flights
of stairs!

Glucose undergoes a sequence of 11 reactions, each catalyzed by a specific
enzyme. It is converted first to pyruvic acid and then to acetyl CoA. Other sugars,
such as fructose and galactose, also enter the glycolytic sequence (but at different
points) and are converted to pyruvic acid and acetyl CoA.

The series of glycolytic reactions begins with the activation of glucose, its
conversion to glucose-6-phosphate in a reaction catalyzed by hexokinase or glucokinase. Hexokinase is present in most, if not all, tissues of the human and has
a high affinity for hexoses (its K_m for glucose is 10^{-5} M). It phosphorylates not

only glucose, but also fructose and mannose. Glucokinase is found principally in the liver, which also has a hexokinase; it is highly specific for glucose and has a much higher K_m for glucose (0.01 M) than does hexokinase. Glucokinase probably functions in the liver primarily for the storage of glucose as glycogen when the concentration of glucose in the blood is high.

Glucose-6-phosphate undergoes a rearrangement catalyzed by an isomerase to yield fructose-6-phosphate, which then accepts a second phosphate group from ATP to form fructose-1,6-diphosphate. The enzyme catalyzing this reaction, phosphofructokinase, regulates and limits the overall rate of glycolysis. High concentrations of ATP or citrate inhibit phosphofructokinase by indicating that the supply of energy in the cell is abundant and that the rate of production of energy via glycolysis and the tricarboxylic acid cycle can be decreased. An increased concentration of AMP stimulates phosphofructokinase by indicating that the cell needs more energy, and this increases the rate of the phosphofructokinase reaction.

Fructose-1,6-diphosphate is then split into two three-carbon sugars, glyceraldehyde-3-phosphate and dihydroxyacetone phosphate. Dihydroxyacetone phosphate is readily converted by an isomerase to glyceraldehyde-3-phosphate for further metabolism in glycolysis.

When a neutral fat is cleaved into fatty acids and glycerol, the fatty acids are metabolized to acetyl CoA, but the glycerol enters the glycolytic pathway. Glycerol is activated by reacting with ATP to form glycerol phosphate and ADP. The glycerol phosphate then undergoes a dehydrogenation with NAD as primary acceptor to yield dihydroxyacetone phosphate:

$$\text{Glycerol} + \text{ATP} \rightarrow \text{Glycerol phosphate} + \text{ADP}$$
$$\text{Glycerol phosphate} + \text{NAD}^+ \rightarrow \text{Dihydroxyacetone phosphate} + \text{NADH} + \text{H}^+$$

The dihydroxyacetone phosphate is converted by the isomerase to glyceraldehyde-3-phosphate and continues in the glycolytic pathway.

In the reactions described so far, glucose has been converted to two molecules of glyceraldehyde-3-phosphate. No biologically useful energy has been gained in these reactions; indeed, there has been a loss of energy, for the $\sim$P from two molecules of ATP has been invested in the reactions to date. In the next reactions, the cell begins to harvest some of the energy contained in glyceraldehyde-3-phosphate.

Catalyzed by glyceraldehyde-3-phosphate dehydrogenase, glyceraldehyde-3-phosphate is converted to 1,3-diphosphoglyceric acid:

$$\text{Glyceraldehyde-3-phosphate} + \text{NAD}^+ \text{ P}_i \rightarrow$$
$$\text{1,3-diphosphoglycerate} + \text{NADH} + \text{H}^+$$

The substrate, glyceraldehyde-3-phosphate, reacts with an -SH group in the enzyme,

forming an H-C-OH group that can undergo dehydrogenation with NAD as hydrogen acceptor. The aldehyde group is oxidized to a carboxyl group with the phosphate attached. This is a mixed anhydride, that is, an energy-rich phosphate group. In this oxidation–reduction reaction, an energy-rich phosphate group is generated at the substrate level. The phosphate group at carbon 1 of 1,3-diphosphoglycerate has a high transfer potential; in the next reaction, the phosphate group is transferred to ADP to yield ATP:

$$1,3\text{-Diphosphoglycerate} + \text{ADP} \rightarrow \text{ATP} + 3\text{-Phosphoglycerate}$$

In these two reactions, an aldehyde (glyceraldehyde-3-phosphate) is oxidized to a carboxylic acid (3-phosphoglycerate); NAD^+ is reduced to NADH; and ATP is formed from ADP and inorganic phosphate.

The 3-phosphoglycerate undergoes an intramolecular rearrangement catalyzed by phosphoglyceromutase to 2-phosphoglycerate. Then, in an unusual reaction, an energy-rich phosphate is generated by the removal of water rather than by the removal of hydrogens, a reaction catalyzed by enolase. The product, phosphoenol pyruvate, has a phosphate group with a high phosphate transfer potential and can transfer its phosphate group to ADP to yield ATP and free pyruvic acid:

$$\text{Phosphoenol pyruvate} + \text{ADP} \rightarrow \text{ATP} + \text{Pyruvic acid}$$

This is the second energy-rich phosphate group generated at the substrate level in the metabolism of glyceraldehyde-3-phosphate to pyruvic acid.

Each glucose molecule metabolized yields two molecules of glyceraldehyde-3-phosphate (one from dihydroxyacetone phosphate). Thus a total of four energy-rich phosphates is produced as one molecule of glucose is metabolized to pyruvic acid. However, two $\sim P$ are invested at the beginning of the process, one to convert glucose to glucose-6-phosphate and the second to convert fructose-6-phosphate to fructose-1,6-diphosphate. The *net* yield in the process is two $\sim P$ (four $\sim P$ produced minus two $\sim P$ used in the reaction). The overall reaction is

$$\text{Glucose} + 2\ P_i + 2\ \text{ADP} + 2\ NAD^+ \rightarrow$$
$$2\ \text{Pyruvate} + 2\ \text{ATP} + 2\ \text{NADH} + 2\ H^+ + 2\ H_2O$$

CONVERSION OF PYRUVATE TO ACETYL CoA

The metabolism of pyruvate to acetyl CoA is a complex, multistep reaction catalyzed by an organized assembly of three kinds of enzymes, the pyruvic dehydrogenase complex. This complex, which has been studied especially in *Escherichia coli,* has proved to be a very large assemblage of three kinds of enzymes, a total of 48 polypeptide chains, and a mass of about 4,600,000 daltons. The proximity of the three kinds of enzymes permits the coordinated catalysis of the overall reaction, increases the overall reaction rate, and minimizes the number of side reactions.

As the first step of this complex reaction, pyruvate combines with thiamine pyrophosphate (TPP) and is decarboxylated by pyruvate dehydrogenase, yielding hydroxyethyl TPP. Second, the hydroxyethyl group attached to TPP is oxidized to an acetyl group and transferred to lipoamide. In this reaction, the disulfide group of lipoamide is reduced to the sulfhydryl form. The product of this reaction, catalyzed by dihydrolipoyl transacetylase, is acetyl lipoamide.

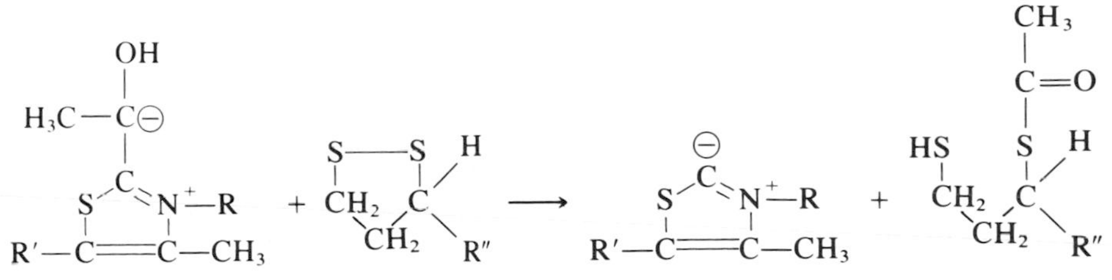

Lipoamide   Acetyl lipoamide

Third, the acetyl group is transferred from acetyl lipoamide to CoA, forming acetyl CoA. This reaction is also catalyzed by dihydrolipoyl transacetylase. The energy-rich thioester bond is conserved as the acetyl group is transferred.

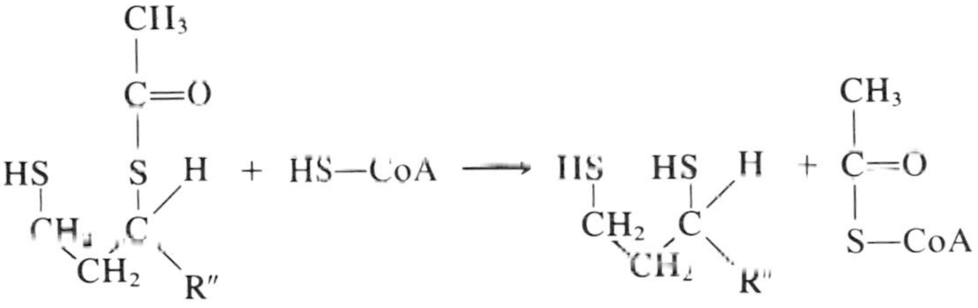

Dihydrolipoamide

Finally, the oxidized form of lipoamide is regenerated in a reaction in which dihydrolipoyl dehydrogenase is the catalyst and NAD^+ accepts the hydrogens removed from dihydrolipoamide. The lipoamide is then ready to react again with hydroxyethyl TPP.

The conversion of pyruvate to acetyl CoA is irreversible, which places some restraints on the patterns of intermediary metabolism. Glucose is not the only source of acetyl CoA, however, nor even quantitatively the most important.

FATTY ACID OXIDATION

The long carbon chain of a saturated fatty acid is split into two-carbon acetyl CoA units by a cyclic sequence of reactions that includes dehydrogenations and make-ready reactions, but not decarboxylations. The overall process is termed *β-oxidation*, since the oxygen atom is added to the *β*-carbon, the second carbon from the carboxyl group. Palmitic acid, a saturated fatty acid with a chain of 16 carbon atoms, is first activated by enzyme-catalyzed reactions with ATP and CoA to form palmityl CoA. This undergoes a dehydrogenation between the second and third carbons of the chain. The group undergoing dehydrogenation is a -CH_2-CH_2- group, and the primary acceptor of the electrons and protons liberated is a flavin. The product, a long-chain molecule with a double bond between carbons 2 and 3, undergoes a make-ready reaction, the addition of a molecule of water across the double bond. The resulting molecule has an H-C-OH group at the β-carbon that can undergo dehydrogenation with NAD as acceptor. The product, a long-chain fatty acid with a C=O group at the β-carbon (carbon 3) and with CoA still attached to its carboxyl carbon, reacts with a second molecule of CoA. The CoA attacks at the C=O group, attaching to it, cleaving off carbons 1 and 2 (with the original CoA group attached) as acetyl CoA, and leaving a carbon chain that is two carbons shorter. This product has CoA attached to its carboxyl group and is ready, without any further activation, to be dehydrogenated by the enzyme that uses flavin as the primary acceptor.

This β-oxidation pathway is a recurring sequence of four reactions:

1. FAD-linked dehydrogenation
2. Hydration
3. NAD-linked dehydrogenation
4. Thiolysis, the cleaving of a molecule by the addition of CoA

Seven such series of dehydrogenations and make-ready reactions split the 16-carbon chain of palmitic acid to eight 2-carbon fragments, each with a CoA group attached, eight acetyl CoAs. The acetyl CoA molecules derived from fatty acid oxidation join those derived from glycolysis and are metabolized further in the tricarboxylic acid cycle.

TRICARBOXYLIC ACID (TCA) CYCLE

Central to the generation of ATP by all human cells, as well as the cells of most lower organisms is the tricarboxylic acid cycle, which begins with the combination of a two-carbon unit (as acetyl CoA) with a four-carbon member of the cycle (oxaloacetic acid) to yield citric acid (six carbons). Citric acid undergoes a remarkable sequence of make-ready reactions, dehydrogenations, and decarboxylations to yield first five-carbon, then four-carbon intermediates that eventually become oxaloacetic acid, ready to combine with another molecule of acetyl CoA. In the course of the cycle, two molecules of carbon dioxide are released, eight protons and electrons are removed, and one molecule of ~P is generated at the substrate level.

Acetyl CoA is derived from the oxidation of fatty acids or from pyruvate formed during glycolysis. The carbon chains of amino acids also enter the tricarboxylic acid cycle, either directly or indirectly via a series of intermediate reactions. Only a small amount of ATP (one $\sim$P) is generated in the TCA cycle itself at the substrate level, just as a small amount of ATP is generated in glycolysis at the substrate level. Most of the cell's ATP is generated by oxidative phosphorylation, by the conversion of ADP to ATP in reactions coupled with the flow of electrons from substrate to oxygen in the electron transport system in the mitochondria. The enzymes catalyzing the reactions of the tricarboxylic acid cycle are also located in the mitochondria, along with the enzymes of the pyruvate dehydrogenase complex. The tidy centralization of these reactions within the mitochondria created some other problems of getting substrates into the mitochondria and transferring the ATP from the mitochondria to the cytosol to be used in driving other reactions.

Acetyl CoA undergoes a make-ready reaction by combining with oxaloacetate to form citrate, plus free CoA. This reaction, an aldol condensation, is catalyzed by citrate synthetase.

$$
\begin{array}{c}
\text{O}{=}\text{C}{-}\text{COO}^- \\
| \\
\text{H}_2\text{C}{-}\text{COO}^-
\end{array}
\quad + \quad
\begin{array}{c}
\text{O} \\
\| \\
\text{CH}_3{-}\text{C} \\
| \\
\text{S}{-}\text{CoA}
\end{array}
\quad \longrightarrow \quad
\begin{array}{c}
\text{CH}_2{-}\text{C}{\overset{O}{\nwarrow}}\text{S}{-}\text{CoA} \\
| \\
\text{C}{-}\text{COO}^- \\
\text{HO}{\diagup}| \\
\text{CH}_2\text{COO}^-
\end{array}
\quad \xrightarrow{\text{H}_2\text{O}}
$$

Oxaloacetate   Citryl CoA

$$
\begin{array}{c}
\text{CH}_2{-}\text{COO}^- \\
| \\
\text{HOC}{-}\text{COO}^- \\
| \\
\text{CH}_2{-}\text{COO}^-
\end{array}
\quad + \quad \text{HS}{-}\text{CoA} + \text{H}^+
$$

The initial product, citryl CoA, is hydrolyzed by the enzyme to citrate and free CoA; the hydrolysis of the citryl CoA pulls the overall reaction in the direction of citrate synthesis. Citrate has neither an H-$\overset{|}{\underset{|}{\text{C}}}$-OH group nor a -CH$_2$-CH$_2$- group and cannot undergo dehydrogenation. Two further make-ready reactions, involving the removal and addition of a molecule of water, yield isocitrate, which can undergo dehydrogenation at its H-C-OH group. The dehydration and hydration reactions are catalyzed by aconitase.

$$
\begin{array}{c}
\text{H}_2\text{C}{-}\text{COO}^- \\
| \\
\text{HO}{-}\text{C}{-}\text{COO}^- \\
| \\
\text{H}_2\text{C}{-}\text{COO}^-
\end{array}
\quad \xrightarrow{-\text{H}_2\text{O}} \quad
\begin{array}{c}
\text{H}_2{\cdot}\text{C}{-}\text{COO}^- \\
| \\
\text{C}{-}\text{COO}^- \\
\| \\
\text{HC}{-}\text{COO}^-
\end{array}
\quad \xrightarrow{+\text{H}_2\text{O}} \quad
\begin{array}{c}
\text{H}_2{\cdot}\text{C}{-}\text{COO}^- \\
| \\
\text{H}{\cdot}\text{C}{-}\text{COO}^- \\
| \\
\text{HO}{\cdot}\text{C}{\cdot}\text{COO}^- \\
\text{H}
\end{array}
$$

Citrate

Isocitrate

The oxidative decarboxylation of isocitrate is catalyzed by isocitrate dehydrogenase. One form of this enzyme, which is located in the mitochondria and uses NAD^+ specifically as hydrogen acceptor, is part of the tricarboxylic acid cycle. A second form of the enzyme, which is located in the cytosol and uses $NADP^+$ as hydrogen acceptor, generates NADPH, which is used as a hydrogen donor in several kinds of biosynthetic reactions. The product of dehydrogenation, oxalosuccinate, undergoes decarboxylation while bound to the enzyme and yields α-ketoglutarate.

$$
\begin{array}{c}
H_2C\cdot COO^- \\
| \\
H\cdot C\cdot COO^- \\
| \\
HO\cdot C\cdot COO^- \\
| \\
H
\end{array}
\xrightarrow[]{NAD^+ \quad NADH + H^+}
\begin{array}{c}
H_2C\cdot COO^- \\
| \\
HC\cdot COO^- \\
| \\
O{=}C\cdot COO^-
\end{array}
\xrightarrow[CO_2]{H}
\begin{array}{c}
H_2C\cdot COO^- \\
| \\
HCH \\
| \\
O{=}C\cdot COO^-
\end{array}
$$

Oxalosuccinate α-Ketoglutarate

The oxidative decarboxylation of α-ketoglutarate yields succinyl CoA. Just as pyruvate is converted to the CoA derivative of an acid with one less carbon atom (acetyl CoA), α-ketoglutarate (five carbons) is converted to succinyl CoA (four carbons) by a similar complex of three kinds of enzymes involving as coenzymes not only NAD^+ and CoA, but also TPP, lipoamide, and FAD.

$$\alpha\text{-ketoglutarate} + NAD^+ + CoA \rightarrow \text{Succinyl CoA} + CO_2 + NADH$$

The bond joining CoA to succinate is an energy-rich one with a ΔG^0 of $-8,000$ calories/mol, comparable to that of ATP ($\sim -7,300$ calories/mol). The energy of the bond of acetyl CoA was used in attaching the acetyl group to oxaloacetate. The cleavage of the thioester bond of succinyl CoA can be coupled to the phosphorylation of guanosine diphosphate (GDP), catalyzed by succinyl CoA synthetase, to yield guanosine triphosphate (GTP):

$$\text{Succinyl CoA} + P_i + GDP \rightarrow \text{Succinate} + GTP + \text{CoA-SH}$$

The phosphoryl group of GTP can then be transferred to ADP to form ATP, a reaction catalyzed by nucleoside diphosphokinase.

$$GTP + ADP \rightarrow GDP + ATP$$

This is a second example of an energy-rich bond generated at the substrate level by reactions not involving the electron transport system. This is the only reaction in the tricarboxylic acid cycle that yields an energy-rich phosphate bond directly; the rest of the ATP is generated by oxidative phosphorylation, coupled to the flow of electrons through the electron transport system in the mitochondria.

The final portion of the tricarboxylic acid cycle involves reactions of four-carbon dicarboxylic acids, succinate, fumarate, malate, and oxaloacetate. The dehydrogenation of succinate, with a $-CH_2-CH_2-$ configuration, involves a flavin as hydrogen and electron acceptor. Succinic dehydrogenase catalyzes the conversion of succinate to fumarate; the hydrogens removed from succinate are transferred to FAD, forming $FADH_2$. The FAD is covalently attached to a histidine residue in the peptide chain of the enzyme. Succinic dehydrogenase contains four atoms of iron and four inorganic sulfides, but no heme group; the iron atoms are probably bonded to the inorganic sulfides; thus succinic dehydrogenase is an example of a "non-heme" iron protein. Unlike other enzymes of the tricarboxylic acid cycle, succinic dehydrogenase is an integral part of the inner mitochondrial membrane and is linked directly to the electron transport system. The $FADH_2$ produced by the dehydrogenation of succinate does not dissociate from the enzyme, but transfers two electrons to the Fe^{3+} atoms of the enzyme.

$$
\begin{array}{ccccccc}
\text{COO}^- & & \text{COO}^- & & \text{COO}^- & & \text{COO}^- \\
| & \text{FAD } \text{FADH}_2 & | & & | & \text{NADH} & | \\
\text{CH}_2 & \xrightarrow{\qquad} & \text{CH} & + \text{H}_2\text{O} & \text{H·C·OH} & \text{NAD}^+ \quad \text{H}^+ & \text{C}{=}\text{O} \\
| & & \| & & | & \xrightarrow{\qquad} & | \\
\text{CH}_2 & & \text{CH} & & \text{H·C·H} & & \text{CH}_2 \\
| & & | & & | & & | \\
\text{COO}^- & & \text{COO}^- & & \text{COO}^- & & \text{COO}^- \\
\text{Succinate} & & \text{Fumarate} & & \text{Malate} & & \text{Oxaloacetate}
\end{array}
$$

Fumarate undergoes a make-ready reaction, the addition of a molecule of water across the double bond, to yield malate. Fumarase catalyzes a stereospecific *trans* addition of H and OH to form the L-isomer of malate. Malate has an

H-C-OH configuration and can undergo dehydrogenation by malate dehydrogenase,

which uses NAD^+ as hydrogen acceptor and yields oxaloacetate, completing the cycle. Even though the oxidation of malate is endergonic, with a ΔG^0 of $+7,000$ calories/mol, the reaction can proceed because the concentrations of the products are very low under physiologic conditions. Both oxaloacetate and NADH are rapidly converted to other products by exergonic reactions. Oxaloacetate may undergo several reactions in addition to its condensation with acetyl CoA to yield citrate, for example, transamination to aspartate and decarboxylation to pyruvate.

This cycle of reactions, which was first described by the English biochemist, Sir Hans Krebs, is usually called the Krebs cycle. By studying the factors that increase the rate at which oxygen is used by slices or minces of kidney, liver and muscle, Krebs, Szent–Györgyi, Martius, and Knoop each contributed critical observations about substances that acted "catalytically"—that increased the uptake of oxygen far more than could be accounted for by their direct oxidation. Finally, Krebs observed that citrate was accumulated by muscle suspensions if oxaloacetate was added. In 1937, Krebs put these findings together in a conceptual framework and postulated the cyclic series of reactions.

The overall reaction of the TCA cycle is:

Acetyl CoA + 3 NAD^+ + FAD + GDP + P_i + 2 H_2O →

$\qquad\qquad$ 2 CO_2 + 3 NADH + $FADH_2$ + GTP + 2 H^+ + CoA

Two carbon atoms enter the cycle as acetyl CoA condenses with oxaloacetate. Two carbon atoms leave the cycle as carbon dioxide in the decarboxylations catalyzed by isocitrate dehydrogenase and α-ketoglutarate dehydrogenase. The two carbons that leave the cycle as carbon dioxide entered the cycle in oxaloacetate, however, not acetyl CoA. Four pairs of hydrogen atoms leave the cycle, three as NADH in the reactions catalyzed by isocitrate dehydrogenase, α-ketoglutarate dehydrogenase, and malate dehydrogenase and one as $FADH_2$ in the reaction catalyzed by succinic dehydrogenase. One energy-rich phosphate is generated as GTP from the energy-rich thioester bond of succinyl CoA, and 2 mol water enter the cycle, one in the synthesis of citrate and the other in the hydration of fumarate. The transfer of electrons to oxygen through the electron transport system generates three ATPs for each pair of electrons from NADH and two ATPs for each pair of electrons from $FADH_2$. Thus a total of 11 energy-rich phosphate bonds are generated when the electrons from three NADH and one $FADH_2$ flow through the electron transport system to oxygen. These, plus the ATP generated at the substrate level from succinyl CoA, make a total of 12 ATPs generated by the complete oxidation of 1 mol acetyl CoA.

The rate of the tricarboxylic acid cycle is regulated to meet the cell's needs for ATP. The synthesis of citrate from oxaloacetate and acetyl CoA is inhibited by ATP so that less ATP is produced when the level of ATP is high. Isocitrate dehydrogenase is stimulated by ADP so that, as ATP is used in cellular processes and converted to ADP, the rise in the level of ADP increases the rate of production of ATP. The third control is the level of α-ketoglutarate dehydrogenase, which is inhibited by its products, succinyl CoA and NADH. Thus, by several mechanisms, the entry of acetyl CoA into the cycle and the overall rate of the cycle are decreased when the cell has a high concentration of ATP. When the concentration of ATP falls (and the concentration of ADP rises), the tricarboxylic acid cycle is activated.

BIOLOGIC OXIDATION AND OXIDATIVE PHOSPHORYLATION

An oxidation is defined chemically as a process in which electrons are removed from an atom or molecule; the reverse process, a reduction, is one in which electrons are added to an atom or molecule. In the reversible reaction

$$Fe^{2+} \rightleftarrows Fe^{3+} + e^-$$

the reaction to the right is an oxidation (the removal of an electron) and the reaction to the left is a reduction (the addition of an electron). Every oxidation reaction must be accompanied by a reduction; electrons do not exist in the free state. Living cells obtain biologically useful energy by enzymatic reactions in which electrons flow from one energy level to another, pass from substrate molecules to primary acceptors through the electron transport system, and ultimately react with oxygen and hydrogen ions to form water. NADH and $FADH_2$ have a pair of electrons with a high energy transfer potential; a large amount of energy is released when the electrons are transferred to oxygen. In oxidative phosphorylation, some of this energy is conserved as energy-rich bonds of ATP. In other words, the electron transfer potential of NADH or $FADH_2$ is converted into the phosphate transfer potential of ATP.

In oxidation–reduction reactions, the free energy change is proportional to the tendency of the reactants to donate or accept electrons, expressed numerically as the redox (reduction–oxidation) potential. A substance that can exist in both an oxidized form (e.g., NAD^+) and a reduced form (NADH) is termed a redox couple. The redox potential of a redox couple can be determined by measuring the electromotive force generated by a sample half cell connected to a standard reference half cell, a hydrogen electrode, which at pH 0 is designated as 0.0 volts. The sample half cell consists of an electrode immersed in 1 M H^+ that is in equilibrium with hydrogen gas at 1 atm pressure. The electrodes are connected to a voltmeter, and the half cells are connected by an agar bridge to provide electrical continuity. Electrons flow from one half cell to another, and the redox potential (E_0) of the NAD^+–NADH couple is the observed voltage at the beginning of the experiment, when the concentrations of NAD^+, NADH, and H^+ are all 1 M. For biologic systems, it is customary to express the redox potential E_0' at pH 7.0 at which pH the E_0' of the hydrogen electrode is -0.42 volts.

The redox potential describes the affinity of a substance for electrons. A negative redox potential means that the substance has a lower affinity for electrons than does H_2. Such substances readily donate electrons to other compounds. A positive redox potential means that the substance has a higher affinity for electrons than does H_2. A strong reducing agent, such as NADH, has a weak affinity for electrons and a negative redox potential, whereas oxygen, a strong oxidizing agent, has a strong affinity for electrons and a positive redox potential.

The redox potentials of many biologically important compounds have been measured. From the difference in the redox potentials of the reactants, it is possible to calculate the free energy change of an oxidation–reduction reaction. In the reduction of oxaloacetate by NADH, for example,

$$\text{Oxaloacetate} + \text{NADH} + H^+ \rightleftharpoons \text{Malate} + NAD^+$$

the redox potential of the NAD^+–NADH couple determined experimentally is -0.32 V and of oxaloacetate–malate is -0.17 V. By convention, oxidation–reduction reactions are written as oxidant + e^- → reductant:

$$\text{Oxaloacetate} + 2 H^+ + 2 e^- \rightarrow \text{Malate}, \ E_0' = -0.17 \text{ V}$$

$$NAD^+ + H^+ + 2 e^- \rightarrow \text{NADH}, \ E_0' = -0.32 \text{ V}$$

Subtracting the second partial reaction from the first yields the overall reduction of oxaloacetate by NADH and a $\Delta E_0'$ of $+0.15$ V. The standard free energy change, ΔG^0, can be calculated from the change in redox potential by the equation

$$\Delta G^0 = -nF\Delta E_0'$$

where n is the number of electrons transferred (two in this reaction), F is the caloric equivalent of the faraday (23,040 calories/V), $\Delta E_0'$ is in volts and ΔG^0 is expressed in calories/mol. For the reduction of oxaloacetate,

$$\Delta G^0 = -2 \times 23{,}040 \times 0.15, \text{ or } -6{,}912 \text{ calories/mol}$$

A positive value for $\Delta E_0'$, as in this equation, signifies an exergonic reaction and yields a negative value for ΔG^0. The value of $\Delta E_0'$ applies to reactions occurring at a pH of 7. Reactions within the cell occur at a pH closer to 7.4, however. Since the standard potential of any half reaction involving a proton, H^+, is pH-dependent, a small correction in the standard value for the redox potential is required.

A complex system of coupled enzymes within the mitochondria carries out the transfer of electrons involved in the oxidation of NADH (or $FADH_2$) by molecular oxygen. The partial reactions involved are

$$\tfrac{1}{2} O_2 + 2\,H^+ + 2\,e^- \rightarrow H_2O \qquad E_0' = +0.82 \text{ V}$$

$$NAD^+ + H^+ + 2\,e^- \rightarrow NADH \quad E_0' = -0.32 \text{ V}$$

Subtracting the second from the first gives

$$\tfrac{1}{2}O_2 + NADH + H^+ \rightarrow H_2O + NAD^+ \quad \Delta E_0' = +1.14 \text{ V.}$$

Thus the change in free energy of this overall reaction is

$$\Delta\,G^0 = -nF\Delta E_0' = -2 \times 23{,}040 \times 1.14 = -52{,}530 \text{ calories/mol}$$

RESPIRATORY CHAIN

The series of catalysts called the respiratory chain include flavin, quinone, and heme groups; these are concerned with the transfer of reducing equivalents, hydrogen ions, and electrons, and with the reaction of these reducing equivalents with oxygen. Some of these catalysts are the prosthetic groups of proteins. The components of the respiratory chain can be arranged in the order of their increasing redox potentials, since electrons flow through the respiratory chain in a stepwise fashion from the more electronegative components to the more electropositive ones and, finally, to oxygen.

At the substrate (electronegative) end of the chain, dehydrogenases catalyze the transfer of electrons from the substrate (e.g., lactate) to NAD, reducing it to NADH. The NADH in turn is oxidized by a metalloflavoprotein enzyme, NADH dehydrogenase. This enzyme contains non-heme iron and flavin mononucleotide (FMN) tightly bound as a prosthetic group. Two electrons are transferred from NADH to FMN, yielding NAD^+ and $FMNH_2$. Electrons then pass from the $FMNH_2$ portion of the NADH dehydrogenase to coenzyme Q, reducing it. Coenzyme Q (also called ubiquinone) is a constituent of the mitochondrial lipids and has a structure similar to that of vitamins K and E, with a long isoprenoid tail.

This tail renders coenzyme Q very nonpolar and readily soluble in the nonaqueous phase of the mitochondrial inner membrane. Coenzyme Q serves as a mobile carrier of electrons between the flavoproteins and the cytochromes. The electrons of $FADH_2$ formed by the action of succinic dehydrogenase are also transferred to coenzyme Q for entry into the cytochrome system.

The cytochromes, electron-transporting proteins that contain a heme prosthetic group, are carriers of electrons from coenzyme Q to oxygen. The iron atom in the heme of the cytochromes alternates between a reduced ferrous (Fe^{2+}) state and an oxidized ferric (Fe^{3+}) state during electron transport. Each heme group carries one electron (in contrast to NADH, the flavins, and coenzyme Q, all of which carry two electrons). Each molecule of reduced coenzyme Q must transfer its two electrons to two molecules of cytochrome b, the next member of the electron transport system.

Five cytochromes with sequentially increasing redox potentials and distinctive structures and properties transport electrons from coenzyme Q to oxygen: cytochromes b, c_1, c, a, and a_3. The heme group of cytochromes b, c_1 and c is iron protoporphyrin IX, and that of cytochromes a and a_3 is an iron porphyrin group, heme A, with slightly different side chains. In cytochromes c and c_1, the heme is attached by thioether bonds to cysteine residues in the peptide chain. Cytochromes a and a_3 exist as a complex, cytochrome oxidase. Electrons are first transferred to the cytochrome a portion of the complex and then to cytochrome a_3, which contains copper. The copper atom is changed from a Cu^{1+} form to a Cu^{2+} oxidized form as it transfers electrons to molecular oxygen. To form a molecule of water, four electrons, four protons, and a molecule of oxygen must converge; the means of accomplishing this is unknown.

The several components of the respiratory chain are present in the mitochondria in nearly constant molar proportions. Many of the components appear to be structurally integrated with the inner membrane of the mitochondrion and it is believed that the several components of the respiratory chain have a definite spatial orientation in the inner mitochondrial membrane.

As electrons flow through the electron transport system from NADH to oxygen, ATP is formed at three sites: 1) between NADH and coenzyme Q, 2) between cytochrome b and cytochrome c, and 3) between cytochrome c and oxygen. There must be a difference in redox potential of approximately 0.2 V (or a free energy change of about 9,000 calories) between the components in the respiratory chain to provide enough energy to generate an energy-rich phosphate (approximately 7,000 calories). Four sites in the respiratory chain have such a change— the three listed and the site between flavoprotein and cytochrome b.

The actual sites have been identified by experiments with specific inhibitors. Rotenone inhibits electron transfer from NADH dehydrogenase to coenzyme Q and prevents the synthesis of ATP at site 1. It does not inhibit oxidative phosphorylation with succinate as substrate, however, for these electrons enter the chain at coenzyme Q, beyond the blocked point. As shown by Britton Chance in some elegant spectroscopic experiments, each carrier's oxidized and reduced forms have distinctive absorption spectra. The addition of one of these inhibitors changes the proportion of oxidized and reduced forms of each carrier. For example, the addition of antimycin A increases the reduction of the carriers between NADH and cytochrome b and increases the oxidation of those between cytochrome c and oxygen. Chance concluded that antimycin inhibits the transfer of electrons from cytochrome b to cytochrome c_1, preventing the synthesis of ATP at site 2. In an antimycin-inhibited system, the addition of ascorbate, which directly reduces cytochrome c, permits the passage of electrons from cytochrome c to oxygen and the synthesis of ATP at site 3. Electron flow from cytochrome oxidase to oxygen can be inhibited by cyanide, azide, or carbon monoxide. Cyanide and azide react with the ferric form of the carrier, and carbon monoxide inhibits the ferrous form. With electron flow blocked, ATP cannot be synthesized at site 3.

Further insights into the sites and mechanism of oxidative phosphorylation have come from studies of submitochondrial particles and reconstituted mitochondrial membranes by Ephraim Racker. Mitochondria fragmented into submitochondrial particles by sonic oscillation can carry out oxidative phosphorylation. Electron micrographs show that these particles have large spherical projections on their surface, termed F_1. These projections can be removed by treatment with urea, after which the submitochondrial particle can transfer electrons through the electron transport system, but cannot form ATP. The addition of F_1 projections, termed *coupling factor,* restores the ability of the submitochondrial particles to form ATP as electrons pass through the system. Isolated molecules of F_1 have ATPase activity, which suggests that the reaction catalyzed by F_1 in the intact system is the reverse, the synthesis of ATP. In other experiments, purified isolated cytochrome c and cytochrome oxidase (a plus a_3) were combined with F_1 and certain other coupling factors into synthetic phospholipid vesicles. This reconstituted system carried out phosphorylation at site 3, between cytochrome c and oxygen.

Shuttles Across the Mitochrondrial Membrane

Although much of the NADH oxidized in the electron transport system is generated within the mitochondria by the enzymes of the tricarboxylic acid cycle and by the β-oxidation of fatty acids, some of the reducing equivalents are generated in the cytoplasm (outside the mitochondria) in the dehydrogenations of glycolysis. Intact mitochondria are impermeable to both NAD^+ and NADH. Therefore, the oxidation of NADH generated in the cytoplasm and the regeneration of NAD^+ in the cytosol so that glycolysis can continue are carried out by the passage of the *electrons* from NADH, rather than NADH itself, across the mitochondrial membrane. The electrons are not free, of course, but are incorporated into carriers.

One major carrier is glycerol-3-phosphate, which readily crosses the mitochondrial membrane. In the cytoplasm, NADH reacts with dihydroxyacetone phosphate to form glycerol-3-phosphate and NAD^+, catalyzed by glycerol-3-phosphate dehydrogenase. The glycerol-3-phosphate enters the mitochondria and is reoxidized to dihydroxyacetone phosphate by a mitochondrial glycerol-3-phosphate dehydrogenase that has an FAD prosthetic group. The dihydroxyacetone phosphate formed in this reaction diffuses back out of the mitochondria to the cytosol and becomes available for another round of the shuttle. In the overall reaction, electrons from NADH in the cytosol are converted into electrons bound to $FADH_2$ within the mitochondria.

The $FADH_2$ within the mitochondria transfers its electrons to the respiratory chain at the level of coenzyme Q, like the electrons from succinic dehydrogenase, and hence two rather than three energy-rich phosphates are formed when cytoplasmic NADH is oxidized by the respiratory chain. Although this may seem to waste an energy-rich phosphate, the concentration of NADH inside the mitochondria is greater than that in the cytosol and electrons would tend to flow *out* of the mitochondria if both cytosol and mitochondrial glycerol-3-phosphate dehydrogenases used NAD. The fact that the mitochondrial enzyme is FAD-linked permits electrons from cytoplasmic NADH to pass into the mitochondria against an NADH concentration gradient. The energy required to drive the transport is reflected in this price of one $\sim P$ per two electrons transferred into the mitochondria. It also follows that the total $\sim P$ produced by the complete oxidation of 1 mol glucose is 36 rather than 38. The NADH and $FADH_2$ produced in the oxidation of fatty acids are formed within the mitochondria and can pass electrons directly to the electron transport system.

Another shuttle system involving the diffusion of malate into the mitochondria and the diffusion of aspartic acid out of the mitochondria transports electrons into the mitochondria of heart and liver cells. Unlike the glycerol phosphate shuttle this malate shuttle is readily reversible, and no energy is used in transferring electrons into the mitochondria.

Neither ADP nor ATP can pass freely across the inner mitochondrial membrane. In order to permit ATP, a highly charged polar molecule generated largely within the mitochondria, to reach the cytosol, where most of the cellular utilization of ATP occurs, the inner membrane contains a specific carrier. The flow of ADP into and ATP out of the mitochondria is mediated by the enzyme, ATP–ADP translocase, which makes up about 6% of the protein in the inner mitochondrial membrane. The transports of ADP and ATP are coupled; that is, an ADP can enter only if an ATP exits. Both ADP and ATP pass down their respective concentration gradients, and no energy is required to drive the transport process.

This coupled flow of ADP and ATP, an example of a facilitated exchange diffusion, can be inhibited by a plant poison, atractyloside. Oxidative phosphorylation soon ceases in a cell poisoned with atractyloside, because the supply of ADP within the mitochondria cannot be replenished and all the adenylic nucleotide within the mitochondria has been converted to ATP, which cannot exit.

Because long-chain fatty acids, such as palmitic acid, cannot diffuse across the inner mitochondrial membrane to reach the matrix that contains the fatty acid oxidizing enzymes, a special transport system has evolved for this transfer. Fatty acids are activated (i.e., converted to the fatty acid–CoA compound) by enzymes located outside the mitochondria. Another enzyme transfers the fatty acyl group from CoA to a special carrier molecule, carnitine. Derived from the amino acid lysine, carnitine is 3-hydroxy, 4-trimethyl amino butyrate. The fatty acyl carnitine diffuses readily across the inner mitochondrial membrane. Within the matrix, the fatty acyl group is transferred from carnitine back to CoA, and fatty acid oxidation can proceed. The carnitine diffuses back to the cytoplasmic compartment and is available to combine with another molecule of fatty acid.

Respiratory Control

In the normal, intact cell, the transfer of electrons through the respiratory chain is tightly coupled to phosphorylation; that is, electrons do not flow through the electron transport system unless ADP is phosphorylated to ATP. Oxidative phosphorylation thus requires a source of electrons in some electronegative compound such as NADH, ADP, inorganic phosphate, and oxygen. The concentration of ADP within the cell, indeed within the mitochondrion, determines the rate of oxidative phosphorylation. This can be readily demonstrated by adding ADP to a tissue homogenate and noting the marked increase in oxygen consumption. The rate of oxygen consumption returns to the initial value when the added ADP has been converted to ATP.

This regulation of the rate of oxidative phosphorylation by the concentration of ADP, termed respiratory control, is of great physiologic significance. When the cell does work of some sort and ATP is consumed, the concentration of ADP increases and oxidative phosphorylation increases. Thus the rate of oxidative phosphorylation is regulated by the rate of utilization of ATP. Electrons flow from substrate molecules to oxygen only when ATP must be synthesized, as signaled by the increased concentration of ADP.

The normal coupling of electron flow and the phosphorylation of ADP can be disrupted by 2,4-dinitrophenol and certain other aromatic compounds. In the presence of 2,4-dinitrophenol, electrons flow normally from NADH to oxygen, but the respiratory chain does not form ATP. This increases oxidation of NADH and oxygen consumption; the energy is dissipated as heat. The uncoupling of oxidative phosphorylation is used by certain tissues as a means of generating heat to maintain body temperature. For example, the brown adipose tissue found in the newborn human and other mammals is rich in mitochondria specialized for heat generation. The fatty acids that act as uncoupling agents in this tissue are released under the control of epinephrine. The degree of uncoupling in brown adipose tissue is under hormonal control; the mitochondria there can generate either ATP or heat.

In 1964, Lars Ernster and Rolf Luft reported a case of a 36-year-old woman who had suffered since early childhood from some unknown metabolic disorder. Her basal metabolic rate was more than twice the normal rate, but her thyroid function was normal. She was unable to do prolonged physical work, perspired profusely, drank a great deal of water without having increased urine volume, and ate a great deal of food without gaining weight. A muscle biopsy revealed atypical, highly variable mitochondria. Biochemical studies showed that these mitochondria were not under respiratory control; NADH was oxidized even if ADP was not present. With pyruvate or malate as substrates, P/O ratios ($\sim$P made per oxygen atoms consumed) of 1.5 to 2.6 were obtained instead of the normal 3. In this patient, much of the energy of fuel molecules was converted into heat instead of into ATP. The underlying molecular defect in these mitochondria remains unknown.

ENERGY CHANGES IN HUMAN METABOLISM

Since electrons flow from foodstuffs to oxygen, it is possible to calculate the total flow of electrons from the rate of oxygen utilization. The average oxygen utilization by a 70-kg adult male at rest is 264 ml/min. Each oxygen atom requires two electrons (and two protons) to form a molecule of water. These facts indicate that 2.86×10^{22} electrons flow from foodstuffs, via dehydrogenases, primary acceptors, and cytochromes each minute in all the cells of the body:

$$0.264 \text{ liter/min} \div 22.4 \text{ liter/mol} = 0.0118 \text{ mol/min}$$

0.0118 mol O_2/min $\times$ 4 electrons/mol $O_2 \times 6.03 \times 10^{23}$ (Avogadro's number) $= 2.86 \times 10^{22}$ electrons/min. Since an ampere is defined as the flow of 3.76×10^{20} electrons per minute, this flow of electrons amounts to 76 amperes. This is a great deal of current, for an ordinary 100-W light bulb uses just a little less than one ampere.

These electrons are flowing from substrate to oxygen over a potential difference of 1.14 V. Since volts $\times$ amperes = watts, 1.14 V $\times$ 76 amperes = 86.6 W. The human body at rest thus uses energy at about the same rate as a 100-W light bulb, but differs in that a much larger flow of electrons passes through a much smaller voltage change.

A human fetus just before birth, weighing 3.2 kg, uses oxygen at a rate of 13 to 15 ml/min. This can be calculated from the difference in the oxygen content of blood going to the fetus in the umbilical vein and that in the blood coming from the fetus in the umbilical artery (about 8 ml oxygen per 100 ml blood) times the rate of blood flow (about 180 ml/min). This amount of oxygen utilization reflects an electron flow from foodstuffs to oxygen in all the cells of the fetus of 1.43×10^{21} electrons per minute, or 3.8 amperes. The fetus is using 3.8 amperes at 1.14 V, or 4.3 W. This may appear to be a small amount of energy, for a 5-W light bulb is not very bright. When the values are corrected for weight, however, the fetus uses just a bit more energy, 1.34 W/kg (4.3 W/3.2 kg) than the adult, 1.23 W/kg (86.6 W/70 kg).

MECHANISMS OF OXIDATIVE PHOSPHORYLATION: THE CHEMIOSMOTIC THEORY

Although it had long been known that oxidative phosphorylation occurs in the mitochondria and many experiments had shown that the transfer of electrons from NADH to oxygen results in the production of three $\sim$P, just how the $\sim$Ps are synthesized remained a mystery. From the redox potentials of various members of the electron transport system, it was possible to infer where the phosphorylations are coupled. The mitochondrial enzyme that converts ADP and inorganic phosphate to ATP was isolated and characterized. Several theorists suggested that some sort of energy-rich intermediate was formed and transferred its energy to drive the synthesis of ATP, but despite an intensive search in many laboratories, no such intermediate could be discovered.

A very different mechanism, the chemiosmotic hypothesis, was suggested by Peter Mitchell in 1961. This theory has been supported by experimental evidence from many laboratories and Mitchell was awarded a Nobel Prize in 1978. Mitchell proposed that electron transport and ATP synthesis are coupled by a proton gradient across the mitochondrial membrane. According to this model, the stepwise transfer of electrons from NADH or $FADH_2$ through the electron carriers to oxygen pumps protons across the inner mitochondrial membrane and generates a membrane potential in which the cytoplasmic side is positive. Protons are pumped out of the matrix by three kinds of electron transfer complexes, each associated with a particular step in the electron transport system. The protons subsequently flow back to the matrix of the mitochondria through special sites in the inner membrane where the enzyme that synthesizes ATP from ADP and P_i is located. The protons move down a chemical and energy gradient, releasing energy to drive the synthesis of ATP. Thus the proton gradient across the inner mitochondrial membrane couples phosphorylation with oxidation.

The model requires that the various electron transport enzymes must be spatially oriented with respect to the inner and outer faces of the inner mitochondrial membrane so that the carriers can pump protons out of the matrix as they transport electrons. The spatial organization of the ATP-synthesizing enzyme permits it to use the energy of the proton gradient to drive the synthesis of ATP. The model also requires that the inner mitochondrial membrane be impermeable to the flow of protons (except through the special sites where the ATP-synthesizing enzyme is located); otherwise, the system would be short-circuited by the leakage of protons. A wealth of experimental evidence confirms these hypotheses and demonstrates that a proton gradient is generated across the inner mitochondrial membrane as electrons are transported. Certain of the electron carriers are arranged in the membrane in such a way that they pick up protons from the matrix side and release them on the outer side of the inner membrane, thereby establishing the proton gradient across the membrane.

GLUCONEOGENESIS

The synthesis of glucose from noncarbohydrate sources is termed *gluconeogenesis*. In the human, this occurs in the liver primarily and in the kidney cortex to a much smaller extent. At first, this may appear to be simply a reversal of the reactions of glycolysis. There is a general principle in intermediary metabolism, however, that the pathway by which a molecule is synthesized is not identical to the pathway by which it is degraded; the two pathways may have one or more reversible reactions in common, but each has at least one reaction that is unique. Furthermore, the pathways of synthesis and degradation of each compound are controlled by different regulatory enzymes. The pathways are typically regulated in a coordinated, reciprocal fashion so that the stimulation of the biosynthetic pathway is accompanied by the inhibition of the corresponding degradative pathway. In addition, the energy-requiring reactions of biosynthesis are coupled to the energy-yielding cleavage of ATP, making the overall process essentially irreversible.

Humans and animals require a constant supply of glucose, for many tissues (e.g., the brain, erythrocytes, the kidney medulla, and the testes) require glucose from the blood as their sole or major source of energy. The human brain requires more than 120 g glucose per day. Much of the daily glucose requirement is obtained from the sugars and starches in meals, but within a few hours after a meal, the concentration of glucose circulating in the blood decreases as the glucose is taken up by tissues and converted to glycogen in liver and muscle. Liver glycogen is a reservoir of glucose and is readily converted to blood glucose (except in patients with glycogen storage disease), whereas muscle glycogen serves as a source of ATP for muscle contraction. Muscles have little or no glucose-6-phosphatase, and muscle glycogen is not converted to blood glucose. Humans and other animals constantly make glucose from noncarbohydrate precursors, such as lactate, pyruvate, glycerol, many amino acids, and from the intermediates of the tricarboxylic acid cycle.

The central pathway of gluconeogenesis is the conversion of pyruvate to glucose. Seven reactions are common to glycolysis and gluconeogenesis, and all of these are freely reversible. Three steps in glycolysis are essentially irreversible in the synthesis of glucose and must be bypassed in gluconeogenesis by other enzymes catalyzing different reactions.

The conversion of pyruvate to phosphoenol pyruvate cannot occur by the reversal of the pyruvate kinase reaction, for that reaction has a large negative change in standard free energy and is irreversible. The first step in the bypass is the carboxylation of pyruvate to form oxaloacetate, catalyzed by pyruvate carboxylase, a biotin-containing enzyme in the mitochondria:

$$\text{Pyruvate} + CO_2 + \text{ATP} \rightarrow \text{Oxaloacetate} + \text{ADP} + P_i$$

This oxaloacetate is then reduced by mitochondrial malate dehydrogenase, with NADH as hydrogen donor:

$$\text{Oxaloacetate} + \text{NADH} + H^+ \rightarrow \text{Malate} + \text{NAD}^+$$

The malate passes from the mitochondria into the cytosol and is reoxidized to oxaloacetate by the cytosolic malate dehydrogenase:

$$\text{Malate} + \text{NAD}^+ \rightarrow \text{Oxaloacetate} + \text{NADH} + \text{H}^+$$

This oxaloacetate is then converted to phosphoenol pyruvate by the enzyme phosphoenol pyruvate carboxykinase, a reaction in which GTP serves as the donor of the phosphate group:

$$\text{Oxaloacetate} + \text{GTP} \rightarrow \text{Phosphoenol pyruvate} + \text{CO}_2 + \text{GDP}$$

The conversion of pyruvate to phosphoenol pyruvate requires two $\sim$P groups, one from ATP and one from GTP.

The phosphorylation of fructose-6-phosphate to fructose-1,6-diphosphate is the second step that is irreversible and must be bypassed in gluconeogenesis. The enzyme fructose diphosphatase catalyzes the irreversible hydrolysis of the phosphate at carbon 1 and yields fructose-6-phosphate plus inorganic phosphate.

$$\text{Fructose-1,6-diphosphate} + \text{H}_2\text{O} \rightarrow \text{Fructose-6-phosphate} + \text{P}_i$$

The diphosphatase is inhibited by AMP and stimulated by ATP.

The phosphorylation of glucose by hexokinase is also irreversible under conditions in the cell and is bypassed in gluconeogenesis by a different reaction, catalyzed by glucose-6-phosphatase, the hydrolysis of the phosphate ester bond.

$$\text{Glucose-6-phosphate} + \text{H}_2\text{O} \rightarrow \text{Glucose} + \text{P}_i$$

Glucose-6-phosphatase, which requires Mg^{2+}, is present in the liver and kidney, but not in muscle or brain. This enzyme plays a key physiologic role in maintaining the concentration of glucose in the blood between meals, hydrolyzing glucose-6-phosphate derived from gluconeogenesis or from the degradation of glycogen.

Examination of all the reactions from pyruvate to free glucose

$$2 \text{ Pyruvate} + 4 \text{ ATP} + 2 \text{ GTP} + 2 \text{ NADH} + 2 \text{ H}^+ + 4 \text{ H}_2\text{O} \rightarrow$$

$$\text{Glucose} + 2 \text{ NAD}^+ + 4 \text{ ADP} + 2 \text{ GDP} + 6 \text{ P}_i$$

shows that gluconeogenesis requires six energy-rich phosphate bonds to drive the conversion of 2 mol pyruvate to 1 mol glucose. The conversion of glucose to pyruvate in glycolysis yields only two molecules of ATP.

The enzyme that catalyzes the first step in gluconeogenesis, pyruvate carboxylase, is stimulated by acetyl CoA. The concentration of this enzyme builds up within the mitochondria when fatty acids are oxidized; acetyl CoA also inhibits the pyruvate dehydrogenase system. Thus the accumulation of acetyl CoA inhibits the conversion of pyruvate to acetyl CoA and favors its conversion instead to glucose. Furthermore, fructose diphosphatase is inhibited by AMP, whereas phosphofructokinase is stimulated by AMP, but is inhibited by citrate and by ATP. These controls ensure that, when the tricarboxylic acid cycle is amply supplied with substrates (i.e., acetyl CoA and citrate) and when the cell has an adequate supply of ATP, the gluconeogenic pathway is favored and glucose is stored as glycogen.

At those points in the pathways where glycolysis and gluconeogenesis are catalyzed by different enzymes, it is possible that the two reactions could occur simultaneously and lead to a loss of energy. For example, phosphofructokinase catalyzes the phosphorylation of fructose-6-phosphate by ATP in glycolysis, and fructose diphosphatase catalyzes the hydrolysis of fructose-1,6-diphosphate in gluconeogenesis:

$$ATP + Fructose\text{-}6\text{-}phosphate \rightarrow ADP + Fructose\text{-}1,6\text{-}diphosphate$$
$$Fructose\text{-}1,6\text{-}diphosphate + H_2O \rightarrow Fructose\text{-}6\text{-}phosphate + P_i$$

The sum of these two reactions is

$$ATP + H_2O \rightarrow ADP + P_i$$

This is an energy-wasting hydrolysis of ATP that accomplishes no metabolic work. If the two reactions proceed simultaneously at high rates, there is a large loss of energy, appearing as heat. Such cycles have been termed *futile cycles;* under normal circumstances, the reciprocal regulatory mechanisms prevent the development of these cycles. It has been discovered recently, however, that there are situations in which futile cycles occur physiologically and serve as a rapid source of heat, for example, in animals coming out of hibernation and in insects getting ready to fly on a cold day.

GLYCOGEN AND BLOOD GLUCOSE

Carbohydrates cannot be stored within cells in the form of glucose. This small, water-soluble molecule would rapidly diffuse out of the cell, and even a small accumulation of glucose would disturb the osmotic relationships between the cell and its surrounding fluid. Therefore, carbohydrates are stored in the form of large molecules, starch in plants and glycogen in animals, that consist of long chains of glucose units joined by α-glycoside bonds. The molecules of glycogen are highly branched, with α-1,6 linkages. Glycogen is synthesized by essentially all the tissues of the body, but especially in the liver and muscle. The amount of glycogen in the liver is quite variable, for the liver is a labile reserve of carbohydrate. In a well-fed person, as much as 5% of the wet weight of liver may be glycogen. The content of glycogen in skeletal muscles is less variable and is usually about 1.5% of the wet weight.

The synthesis of glycogen begins with glucose-6-phosphate, formed either by the phosphorylation of glucose catalyzed by hexokinase or glucokinase or by gluconeogenesis from glycerol, phosphoenol pyruvate, or some comparable precursor. Glucose-6-phosphate is reversibly converted to glucose-1-phosphate by phosphoglucomutase. The next step is the formation of uridine diphosphoglucose, UDPG, by a reaction with uridine triphosphate (UTP) catalyzed by glucose-1-phosphate uridyl transferase:

$$\text{Glucose-1-phosphate} + \text{UTP} \rightarrow \text{UDP glucose} + \text{PP}_i$$

The pyrophosphate is split by pyrophosphatase, which causes the reaction to proceed to the right. In the next step, the glucose residue of UDP glucose is transferred to a nonreducing end of the branched glycogen molecule. An $\alpha\text{-}1 \rightarrow 4$ bond is established between carbon 1 of the glucose being transferred and carbon 4 of the terminal glucose residue of glycogen:

$$\text{UDP glucose} + (\text{Glucose})_n \rightarrow \text{UDP} + (\text{Glucose})_{n+1}$$

The overall equilibrium of this set of reactions favors glycogen synthesis. A separate glycogen branching enzyme, glycosyl-(4 → 6)-transferase transfers a short fragment (six or seven glucose units long) of the glucose chain to a 6-hydroxyl group of a glucose in the same or a different glycogen chain, thereby establishing a new branch in the glycogen molecule. The large number of nonreducing ends created by the action of this branching enzyme makes glycogen a better substrate for both glycogen synthesis by glycogen synthase and for glycogenolysis by glycogen phosphorylase, both of which act only on free, nonreducing ends of the glycogen molecule.

The breakdown of glycogen is catalyzed by glycogen phosphorylase, present in most if not all types of human tissues, in a reaction in which the terminal glucose in a glycogen chain is removed by the addition of inorganic phosphate (phosphorolysis) to yield glucose-1-phosphate:

$$(\text{Glucose})_n + \text{P}_i \rightarrow \text{Glucose-1-phosphate} + (\text{Glucose})_{n-1}$$

Glycogen phosphorylase can act repeatedly on a glucose chain in glycogen until it reaches a point within four glucose residues of an $\alpha\text{-}(1 \rightarrow 6)$ branch. At this point, another enzyme, $\alpha\text{-}(1 \rightarrow 6)$ glucosidase, takes over, first transferring three of the glucose residues to the nonreducing end of an outer branch, then cleaving off the glucose bound in $\alpha\text{-}(1 \rightarrow 6)$ linkage to yield a molecule of free glucose. This reaction also makes another glucose chain available for attack by glycogen phosphorylase. Glucose-1-phosphate is then converted to glucose-6-phosphate by phosphoglucomutase, and, in the liver and kidney, glucose-6-phosphate is cleaved by glucose-6-phosphatase to yield free glucose and inorganic phosphate.

The major physiologic function of glucose-6-phosphatase is to regulate the concentration of glucose in the blood between meals. The glycogen in the liver, about 80 g, is depleted by a fast of 18 to 24 hours. Glycogenolysis begins approximately 4 hours after a meal to maintain the concentration of glucose in the blood relatively constant. The importance of glucose-6-phosphatase is dramatically demonstrated by glycogen storage disease (von Gierke's disease) in which it is greatly reduced or lacking altogether. The liver accumulates large stores of glycogen, but the patient suffers from severe hypoglycemia if not fed frequently. The repeated bouts of hypoglycemia may cause mental retardation if they are not diagnosed early and treated by frequent feeding and overnight infusion of glucose during sleep.

Other sugars, such as fructose and galactose, enter the glycolytic pathway by reactions in which they are phosphorylated. Fructose may be phosphorylated to fructose-6-phosphate by hexokinase in muscle or kidney; in the liver, however, a separate fructokinase converts it to fructose-1-phosphate, which is cleaved by aldolase, the enzyme that cleaves fructose-1,6-diphosphate. With fructose-1-phosphate, the products are glyceraldehyde and dihydroxyacetone phosphate. The glyceraldehyde is phosphorylated in a reaction with ATP catalyzed by triose kinase, yielding glyceraldehyde-3-phosphate.

The entry of galactose into the glycolytic pathway is a bit more complex. Galactose, a constituent of lactose (the sugar present in milk), is phosphorylated by galactokinase to galactose-1-phosphate, which reacts with UDP glucose in a reaction catalyzed by UDP glucose-galactose-1-phosphate uridylyl transferase to yield UDP galactose and glucose-1-phosphate. While bound to UDP, the galactose moiety is epimerized to yield UDP glucose by the enzyme UDP glucose epimerase. Finally, the UDP glucose is cleaved by UDP glucose pyrophosphorylase to yield glucose-1-phosphate. Galactose is important not only as a food source for infants, but also as a key component of glycoproteins and glycolipids, constituents of cell membranes and cell surfaces.

A genetic defect in which there is no gene for uridylyl transferase causes galactosemia. This lack prevents the overall conversion of galactose to glucose, and galactose-1-phosphate, galactose, and galactitol (formed by the reduction of galactose) accumulate in tissues. This results in an enlarged liver, cataracts in the eyes, and damage to the CNS, leading to mental retardation. If diagnosed promptly after birth, these harmful effects can be avoided by a diet that contains no milk or milk products.

PENTOSE PHOSPHATE PATHWAY

An alternative route for the oxidation of glucose is the pentose phosphate pathway. A series of enzymes, quite independent of those of the glycolytic sequence, act in concert with certain glycolytic enzymes and can account for the complete oxidation of glucose to carbon dioxide. The primary purposes of this pathway in metabolism however, are to provide reducing equivalents for the generation of NADPH used in biosynthetic reactions and to synthesize and dispose of pentoses.

In contrast to glycolysis, the pentose phosphate pathway neither generates nor uses ATP. It begins with the dehydrogenation of glucose-6-phosphate, which has an $\overset{|}{\underset{|}{H-C-OH}}$ group that can undergo dehydrogenation with NADP as hydrogen acceptor in a reaction catalyzed by glucose-6-phosphate dehydrogenase. A make-ready reaction, the addition of water, converts the product to 6-phosphogluconic acid. This also has an H-C-OH group and can undergo dehydrogenation by a second enzyme, 6-phosphogluconate dehydrogenase, which also specifically requires NADP as hydrogen acceptor. The product of this reaction undergoes decarboxylation to yield a five-carbon sugar, ribulose-5-phosphate (a reactant of major importance in photosynthesis). Ribulose-5-phosphate is the source of the pentoses, of ribose and deoxyribose, that are constituents of nucleotides, and of nucleic acids. Ribulose-5-phosphate is converted to ribose-5-phosphate by an isomerase, and the ribose-5-phosphate is used in the synthesis of ribonucleotides and deoxyribonucleotides.

The pentose phosphate pathway plays an important role in human red cells, for the NADPH produced reduces glutathione, which in turn is used to reduce hydrogen peroxide. The NADPH also helps in preventing unsaturated fatty acids in the red cell membrane from reacting with H_2O_2 to form peroxides and in maintaining hemoglobin in the Fe^{2+} state. Both unsaturated fatty acids and hemoglobin are attacked by H_2O_2. In the group of human genetic deficiency diseases in which there is a deficiency of glucose-6-phosphate dehydrogenase, the red cells tend to undergo hemolysis, causing anemia. Patients with this deficiency may exhibit no symptoms unless treated with certain drugs, such as the antimalarial primaquine phosphate. Oxidation of these drugs produces H_2O_2 in amounts that require more NADPH than the defective glucose-6-phosphate dehydrogenase system can provide. The excess H_2O_2 attacks the fatty acids in the membrane, converts hemoglobin to methemoglobin, and leads to hemolysis. The antimalarial drug selectively destroys older red cells. The rapid breakdown of red cells leads not only to anemia, but also to jaundice and black urine caused by the excretion of the breakdown products of hemoglobin.

Because the gene for glucose-6-phosphate dehydrogenase is X linked, the deficiency appears much more frequently in males than in females. The gene is present in about 11% of American black males. Most of these have no symptoms unless treated with primaquine or certain sulfa drugs. Many millions of people in Africa and Asia suffer from this deficiency. The illness brought on by the administration of primaquine to such individuals is severe, but rarely fatal. After approximately 1 week the patient begins to recover and the red cell count returns to normal.

4

The Lipids and Their Metabolism

The neutral fats (triacylglycerols) present in the diet are hydrolyzed in the gut by pancreatic lipase, aided by the detergent action of bile salts secreted by the liver. The products are free fatty acids and monoacylglycerols. Both free fatty acids and monoacylglycerols are emulsified, absorbed, and usually resynthesized to neutral fats within the intestinal cells. The bile salts, which play a key role in the absorption of the fat-soluble vitamins, A, D, E, and K, are reabsorbed and returned to the liver to be reused. Neutral fats are transported in the lymph as chylomicrons, droplets of emulsified triacylglycerols with a hydrophobic coat of phospholipids and proteins. Triacylglycerols from chylomicrons are hydrolyzed by lipoprotein lipase, an enzyme located on the outer surface of fat cells (adipocytes), and released into the blood, where they are bound to serum albumin for transport. They may also be taken up by the adipocytes and converted into triacylglycerols for storage. The chylomicrons, depleted of their triacylglycerols, may then return to the gut to pick up more triacylglycerols for transport.

Triacylglycerols stored within adipocytes are not attacked by lipoprotein lipase, but by a separate, hormone-sensitive lipase located within the adipocyte. Epinephrine stimulates the hormone-sensitive lipase of the adipocyte by a mechanism that is mediated by cyclic adenosine monophosphate (cAMP) and involves the phosphorylation of the inactive enzyme to convert it into the active form. The mechanism is similar to that by which epinephrine or glucagon stimulates glycogen phosphorylase of the liver. When insulin is bound to the surface of the adipocyte, it inhibits the effect of epinephrine and decreases the activity of the hormone-sensitive lipase; thus insulin inhibits lipolysis.

Patients with a genetic deficiency of lipoprotein lipase have a reduced ability to attack chylomicrons, which persist for a long time after a meal rich in fats. The use of triacylglycerols is impaired, and they are deposited in yellow, lipid-filled swellings under the skin.

Fatty acids are metabolized to acetyl coenzyme A (CoA), and glycerol is phosphorylated and oxidized to dihydroxyacetone phosphate to undergo glycolysis (see Chapter 3). Two molecules of acetyl CoA may condense to form acetoacetyl CoA; this loses the CoA to become free acetoacetate, which in turn can be reduced enzymatically to β-hydroxybutyrate or decarboxylated to acetone. Acetoacetate, β-hydroxybutyrate, and acetone are called ketone bodies. These pass in the blood to tissues, such as skeletal and cardiac muscle, where they are taken up and enter the tricarboxylic acid cycle. The ketone bodies are essentially a transport form of acetyl groups, supplying energy to the heart and other peripheral tissues. The concentration of ketone bodies in the blood is normally quite low; in prolonged fasting or in diabetes mellitus, however, the concentration rises markedly, resulting in a condition termed *ketosis,* because the liver forms ketone bodies more rapidly than the peripheral tissues can metabolize them.

BIOSYNTHESIS OF FATTY ACIDS AND FATS

Humans have a large capacity to synthesize and store triacylglycerols. An adult 70-kg male has about 12 kg stored triacylglycerols, enough to supply his energy needs for some 50 days. Any carbohydrates eaten in excess of the body's capacity to metabolize them or store them as glycogen are converted to triacylglycerols and stored in adipose tissue.

The synthesis of fatty acids is catalyzed by a group of enzymes quite different from those involved in their oxidation. The fatty acid–synthesizing enzymes are located in the cytosol, whereas the fatty acid–oxidizing enzymes are located in the mitochondria. Fatty acids are synthesized two carbons at a time, just as they are oxidized two carbons at a time. In order to participate in the synthetic reactions, acetyl CoA must be activated by conversion to the three-carbon malonyl CoA. This reaction occurs in the cytosol. Because acetyl CoA is formed within the mitochondria and acetyl CoA cannot pass through the mitochondrial membrane, an acetyl group "shuttle" transfers acetyl groups across the membrane. This involves the reaction of intramitochondrial acetyl CoA with oxaloacetate to form citrate, the first step in the tricarboxylic acid cycle. Citrate passes through the membrane via a specific transport system and in the cytosol is cleaved by citrate lyase to yield acetyl CoA and oxaloacetate:

$$Citrate + ATP + CoA \rightarrow Acetyl\ CoA + ADP + P_i + Oxaloacetate$$

The oxaloacetate is then reduced to malate, which enters the mitochondria by a specific carrier system and is oxidized to oxaloacetate to complete the shuttle.

The cytosolic acetyl CoA is then carboxylated to malonyl CoA by a complex carboxylase enzyme that contains the vitamin biotin:

$$ATP + Acetyl\ CoA + CO_2 + H_2O \rightarrow Malonyl\ CoA + ADP + P_i + H^+$$

The carboxylation of acetyl CoA is the rate-limiting step in the biosynthesis of fatty acids. The enzyme is allosterically stimulated by citrate. When the concentration of citrate in the mitochondria increases, as when glycolysis is occurring rapidly after the ingestion of carbohydrates, the citrate passes out of the mitochondria and serves both as the precursor of cytosolic acetyl CoA and as the signal for the activation of the carboxylase to make malonyl CoA.

Fatty acid synthesis is catalyzed by an organized complex of seven enzymes, fatty acid synthase, located in the cytosol. The fatty acids undergoing synthesis are bound to a special acyl carrier protein (ACP) that contains a phosphopantetheine group. Pantothenic acid, a vitamin, has an -SH group to which the malonyl CoA is attached. The nascent acyl chain is attached to the -SH group of a cysteine residue in the synthase. In the first two reactions of fatty acid synthesis, the synthase is charged with the proper acyl groups. The acetyl group of acetyl CoA is transferred to the cysteine -SH group, and malonyl CoA is transferred to the phosphopantetheine -SH group. When the synthase has been charged with its two covalently bound acyl groups, located close together on the synthase, the chain lengthening process can begin. The acetyl and malonyl groups condense to form an acetoacetyl group bound to the phosphopantetheine -SH group, and carbon dioxide is released. The acetyl group displaces the free carboxyl carbon of malonyl CoA as carbon dioxide. This is the same carbon that was introduced by the carboxylase. The addition and loss of the carbon dioxide drives the condensation reaction.

The acetoacetyl group bound to the acyl carrier protein is first reduced to hydroxybutyryl-S-acyl carrier protein by hydrogens donated by reduced nicotinamide adenine dinucleotide phosphate (NADPH) and then is dehydrated to yield butenoyl-S-ACP, with a double bond between carbons 2 and 3, $CH_3-CH=CH-CO$ S-ACP. This undergoes a second reduction by NADPH to yield the saturated butyryl -S-ACP. The butyryl group is then transferred from the S-pantotheine to the S-cysteine of the enzyme, and the S-pantotheine is ready to accept another malonyl CoA for the next round of chain-lengthening reactions. Seven such cycles yield palmitoyl -S-ACP, and palmitic acid is freed from the enzyme by hydrolysis. The NADPH required for fatty acid synthesis is generated by the phosphogluconate pathway in the liver and by malate enzyme in adipose tissue:

$$\text{Malate} + \text{NADP}^+ \rightarrow \text{Pyruvate} + CO_2 + \text{NADPH} + H^+$$

Both of these reactions occur in the cytosol, creating a strongly reducing environment there. Clearly, the synthesis and oxidation of fatty acids occur by two completely different systems (Table 4–1).

The product of fatty acid synthase, palmitic acid (16 carbons), is the precursor of other fatty acids. A separate enzyme in the endoplasmic reticulum adds another two-carbon unit from malonyl CoA to palmitoyl-S-ACP, forming stearic acid (18 carbons). Stearic and palmitic acids are converted to oleic and palmitoleic acids with a double bond between carbons 9 and 10. This conversion occurs through

Table 4-1. *Synthesis and Oxidation of Fatty Acids*

	Synthesis	Oxidation
Location within the cell	Cytosol	Mitochondria
Acyl carrier group	Acyl carrier protein	CoA
Active two-carbon unit	Malonyl CoA	Acetyl CoA
Electron donor or acceptor	NADPH	FAD and NAD+
CO_2 involved	Yes	No

reactions involving NADPH and mixed function oxidases that require molecular oxygen and yield water and $NADP^+$:

Palmitoyl CoA + NADPH + H^+ + $O_2 \rightarrow$

Palmitoleyl CoA + $NADP^+$ + 2 H_2O

Although animal tissues can introduce a double bond at the 9, 10 position, they cannot introduce other double bonds closer to the methyl terminal end of the fatty acid. Thus linoleic, with two double bonds at Δ^9 and Δ^{12}, and linolenic, with three double bonds at Δ^9, Δ^{12}, and Δ^{15}, cannot be synthesized by humans and other mammals; they must be obtained in the diet. These are termed *essential fatty acids* (meaning they are essential in the diet). Linoleic can be converted by mammalian tissues to arachidonic acid, a 20-carbon fatty acid with four double bonds at carbons 5, 8, 11, and 14. This is the essential precursor of prostaglandins, thromboxanes, and leukotrienes, important hormonelike regulatory substances.

SYNTHESIS OF TRIACYLGLYCEROLS AND PHOSPHOLIPIDS

Triacylglycerols and phospholipids have common precursors, glycerol phosphate and fatty acyl CoAs, as well as several common biosynthetic reactions. Glycerol phosphate can be formed by the phosphorylation of glycerol by adenosine triphosphate (ATP) or by the reduction of dihydroxyacetone phosphate in a reaction in which NADH serves as hydrogen donor. The fatty acyl CoAs are formed from free fatty acids synthesized within the cell or obtained in the diet. Two fatty acyl groups (as acyl CoA) are added to glycerol phosphate to yield diacylglycerol phosphate (also called phosphatidic acid), releasing CoA. Phosphatidic acid is hydrolyzed to form diacylglycerol, which reacts with a third molecule of fatty acyl CoA to yield triacylglycerol. The formation of each ester bond in the triacylglycerol requires the input of free energy for the conversion of the fatty acids to their CoA derivatives.

Diacylglycerols are also the precursors of membrane phospholipids. Diacylglycerol reacts with cytidine diphosphate ethanolamine or with cytidine diphosphate choline to yield phosphatidyl ethanolamine and phosphatidyl choline, respectively. Ethanolamine is phosphorylated by ATP to yield phosphoethanolamine, which reacts with cytidine triphosphate (CTP) to yield cytidine diphosphate ethanolamine and pyrophosphate (PP_i). The phosphatidyl ethanolamine can accept three methyl groups from 3 mol S-adenosyl methionine to form phosphatidyl choline. Alternatively, cytidine diphosphate choline can be synthesized by the condensation of CTP with phosphocholine, made by the phosphorylation of choline by ATP.

COMPLEX LIPIDS: STRUCTURE AND FUNCTION

Other lipid components of membranes are the sphingolipids—sphingomyelins, cerebrosides, and gangliosides. Sphingolipids are composed of a long-chain fatty acid, the long-chain amino alcohol, sphingosine, and a polar head group containing an -OH, alcohol, group. Sphingomyelins, the most abundant sphingolipids, contain sphingosine, a long-chain fatty acid, and phosphoethanolamine or phosphocholine as the polar head group. They are found in the myelin sheath around certain neurons and in cell membranes. Cerebrosides have glucose or galactose as their polar head group, as well as sphingosine and a long-chain fatty acid. These may also be termed *glycolipids* because of the sugars present. More complex cerebrosides may have as many as four sugar units present: these are typically found in the outer layer of cell membranes. Gangliosides, the most complex sphingolipids, have large polar heads containing four or more sugar units, one of which is *N*-acetylneuraminic acid (sialic acid). Gangliosides, which are most abundant in the cell membranes of the gray matter in the brain, are components of the specific receptor sites on the surface of cell membranes, such as those at the tips of dendrites.

Like other cell constituents, sphingolipids undergo a constant metabolic turnover, being synthesized and degraded by different enzymes. There are several genetic defects in which an enzyme that degrades a sphingolipid is missing; as a result, the sphingolipid accumulates in the brain. For example, the lack of sphingomyelinase results in Niemann–Pick disease and the lack of *N*-acetylhexosaminidase results in Tay–Sachs disease. Such defects cause degeneration of the nervous system, mental retardation, and early death. These and other diseases in which the degradation of sphingolipids and proteoglycans is defective are termed *lysosomal diseases*, because the degradative enzymes are normally contained in the lysosomes, small membrane-bounded cytoplasmic vesicles that contain hydrolytic enzymes.

CHOLESTEROL, BILE ACIDS, AND FAT-SOLUBLE VITAMINS

Biosynthesis of Cholesterol

Another important constituent of certain cell membranes and of plasma lipoproteins is cholesterol, which also serves as the precursor of bile acids and steroid hormones. The biosynthesis of cholesterol begins with the condensation of 2 mol acetyl CoA (two carbons) to form acetoacetyl CoA (four carbons) and the addition of 1 mol acetyl CoA to form β-hydroxy-β-methyl glutaryl CoA (six carbons).

β-Hydroxy-β-methyl glutaryl CoA

Hydroxymethyl glutaryl CoA undergoes an irreversible two-step reduction of a carboxyl group to an alcohol group, with loss of the CoA group to yield mevalonate. This, the committed step in cholesterol synthesis, is catalyzed by hydroxymethyl glutaryl CoA reductase.

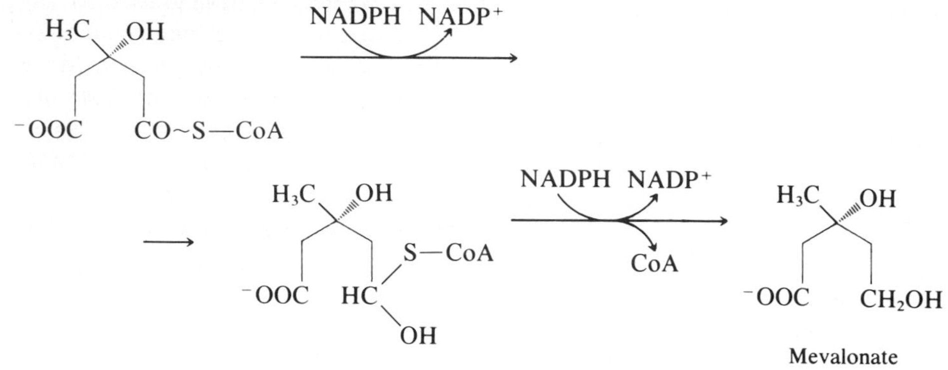

Mevalonate is phosphorylated three times (with 3 mol ATP) to form an unstable compound that undergoes decarboxylation and loses a phosphate to yield isopentenyl pyrophosphate (five carbons). This isomerizes to yield 3,3-dimethyl allyl pyrophosphate. These two isomeric isoprenyl pyrophosphates condense, yielding geranyl pyrophosphate (ten carbons). This reacts with 1 mol isopentenyl pyrophosphate to yield farnesyl pyrophosphate (15 carbons).

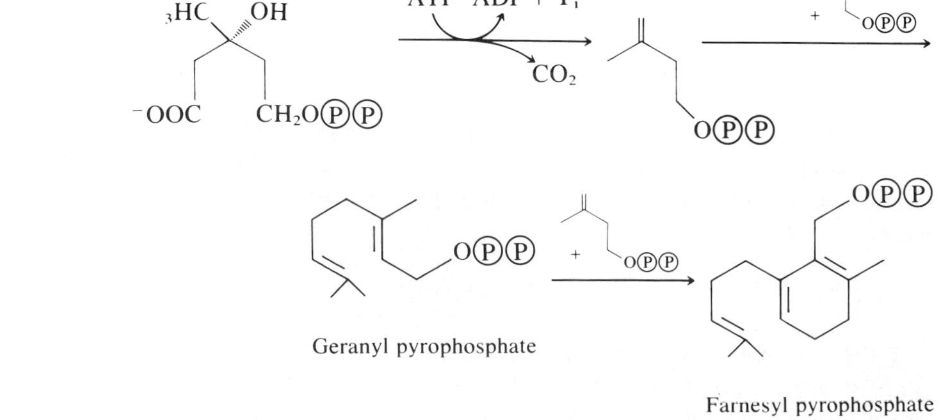

Geranyl pyrophosphate

Farnesyl pyrophosphate

Two molecules of farnesyl pyrophosphate undergo condensation catalyzed by a microsomal enzyme, presqualene synthase, to yield presqualene pyrophosphate

(30 carbons). This is reduced enzymatically with **NADPH** as hydrogen donor to yield squalene (30 carbons) and pyrophosphate.

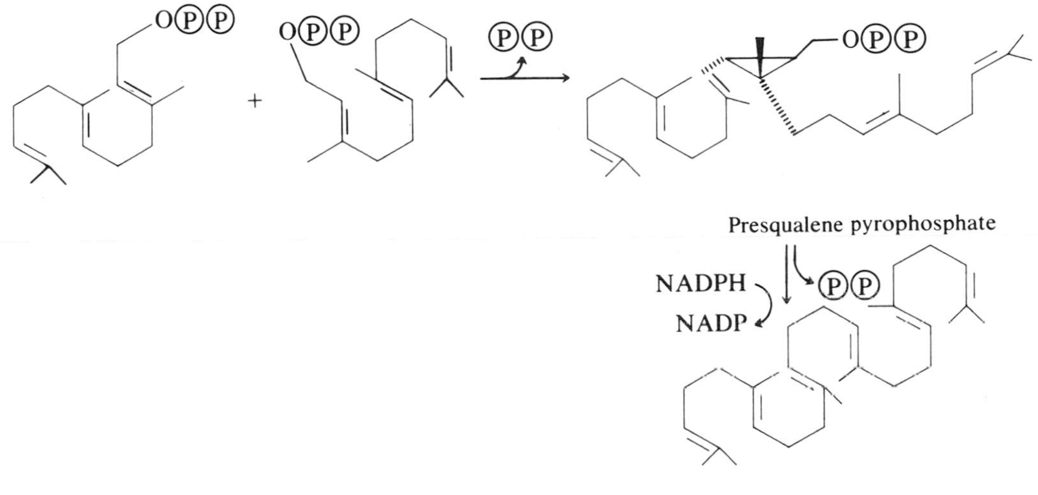

Presqualene pyrophosphate

Squalene

Squalene undergoes a sequence of complex enzymatic reactions in which it is first attacked by molecular oxygen to form squalene-2,3-epoxide; this undergoes cyclization to lanosterol by a series of concerted 1,2 methyl group and hydride shifts along the squalene chain. These bring about the closure of the four rings and require two enzymatic proteins, plus phosphatidyl serine and flavin adenine dinucleotide (FAD).

Squalene-2,3-epoxide

Lanosterol

Lanosterol (30 carbons) is then "pruned" to yield cholesterol (27 carbons). Three angular methyl groups are removed (two from carbon 4 and one from carbon 14). The double bond in the side chain and the double bond between rings B and C are saturated, and a new double bond is inserted between carbons 5 and 6. The sequence of these reactions is not completely fixed; there are several pathways for the conversion of lanosterol to cholesterol. One of these involves 7-dehydrocholesterol, the precursor of vitamin D (cholecalciferol) as the last intermediate.

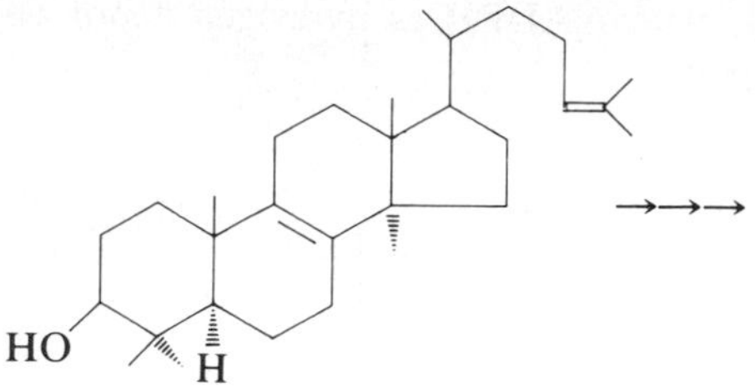

Lanosterol 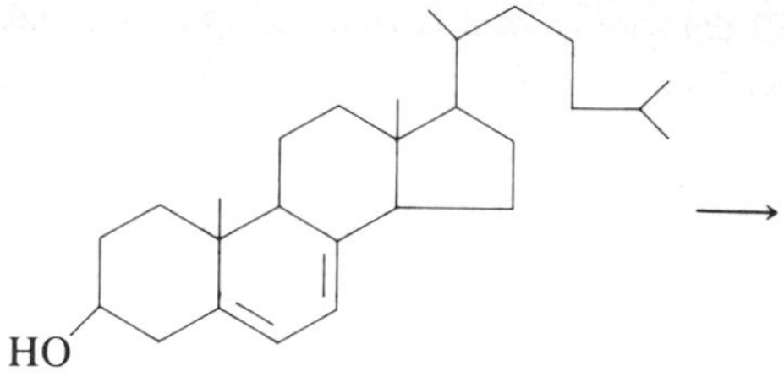   7-Dehydrocholesterol

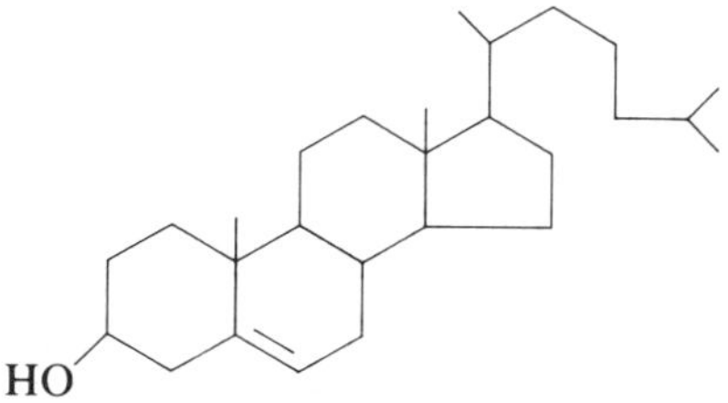

Cholesterol

CONTROL OF CHOLESTEROL BIOSYNTHESIS

A major site of the control of the synthesis of cholesterol is at the committed step, the reduction of β-hydroxy-β-methyl glutaryl CoA to mevalonate, catalyzed by hydroxymethyl glutaryl CoA reductase. Both fasting and the ingestion of cholesterol markedly reduce the activity of and the synthesis of the enzyme in the liver. The activity of the enzyme is increased when an individual resumes feeding after a period of fasting. Increasing the amounts of dietary carbohydrate or triacylglycerol augments cholesterol synthesis from acetyl CoA. Some evidence suggests that dietary cholesterol has a second site of feedback inhibition at the reaction by which squalene is cyclized to lanosterol.

Cholesterol, together with other lipids, may be deposited on the inner walls of blood vessels, a condition termed atherosclerosis. This may lead to the occlusion of blood vessels that supply the heart and the brain, resulting in heart attacks and strokes, respectively. There is still heated discussion as to whether reducing the dietary intake of cholesterol is useful in preventing atherosclerosis and the resulting heart attacks and strokes. If dietary restriction reduced the amount of cholesterol in the blood and in the liver, this would reduce the inhibition of the hydroxymethyl glutaryl CoA reductase and would increase the endogenous synthesis of cholesterol in the liver.

Although the liver is a major site of cholesterol synthesis, other tissues—intestines, adrenal gland, skin, nervous system, aorta, the gonads, and the placenta—also synthesize cholesterol. Cultured human fibroblasts have been used to investigate the control of cholesterol metabolism. Human fibroblasts in culture exhibit a specific cell surface receptor that binds low-density lipoprotein, LDL, the major carrier of cholesterol in plasma. The lipoprotein is bound to the receptor, internalized by endocytosis, and delivered to the lysosomes. The lysosomes degrade the lipoprotein and hydrolyze its cholesterol esters and apoproteins. The free cholesterol enters the cell membranes and represses both the synthesis and the activity of the hydroxymethyl glutaryl CoA reductase.

HYPERCHOLESTEROLEMIA

Familial hypercholesterolemia is a genetically transmitted disorder that is accompanied by high levels of plasma cholesterol and low-density lipoprotein, resulting in premature atherosclerosis. Fibroblasts from such humans have been shown to be deficient in receptors for the plasma low-density lipoprotein. Because of this, the entry of cholesterol esters into the cells is impaired, which eliminates the intracellular feedback on hydroxymethyl gutaryl CoA reductase, that would be exerted by the increased intracellular concentrations of cholesterol. This leads to an unregulated elevated rate of cholesterol synthesis and causes the hypercholesterolemia. Both the heterozygote and the homozygote may show xanthomatosis characterized by multiple benign fatty tumors, called xanthomas, in the skin, tendon sheath, and bone.

A portion of the cholesterol removed from the blood appears in the bile in high concentration. Cholesterol is only very sparingly soluble in water, but it is readily dispersed in aqueous bile in micelles of bile salts and phosphoglycerides. In the gallbladder, water and some of the bile salts are reabsorbed by the mucosa. If continued, this process may remove enough water and bile salts so that cholesterol precipitates as crystals and forms biliary calculi, or gallstones. Calculi may remain in the gallbladder undetected for many years; if they pass down the bile duct and occlude it, however, they may cause severe pain and increase the levels of bile pigments in the serum and tissues, causing jaundice.

Synthesis of Bile Acids

In the human, the major pathway of degradation of cholesterol is its conversion to bile acids. This process involves the hydroxylation of cholesterol at positions 7 and 12, the shortening of the side chain by three carbons, the conversion of the terminal carbon to a carboxyl group, and the formation of the CoA derivative to the carboxyl group to yield cholyl CoA (Fig. 4–1). The condensation of cholyl CoA with glycine or taurine yields glycocholic and taurocholic acid, respectively. These bile salts are very effective detergents and serve in the intestine to make dietary lipids soluble. This promotes hydrolysis by lipases and facilitates their absorption.

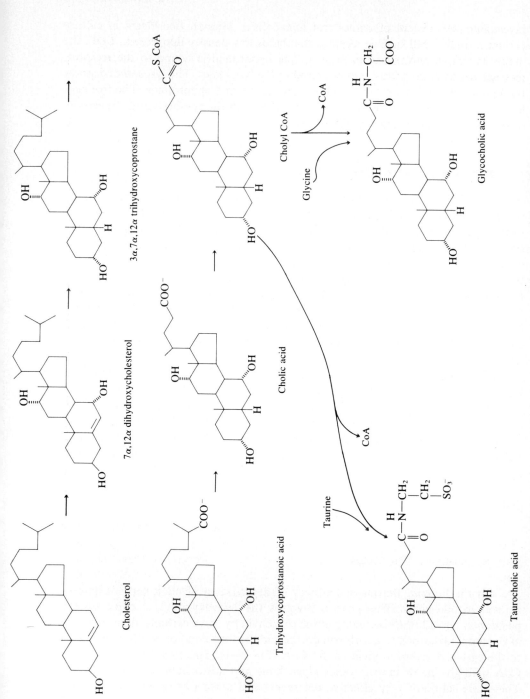

Fig. 4–1. *Synthesis of bile acids, taurocholic acid, and glycocholic acid from cholesterol.*

Fat-Soluble Vitamins

The fat-soluble vitamins A, E, and K, are derivatives of isopentenyl pyrophosphate.

VITAMIN A

Retinol, vitamin A, is composed of four isoprenoid units (dotted lines indicate the junctions of the isoprenoid units).

Plants synthesize from isopentenyl pyrophosphate the 40-carbon compound, β-carotene, which can be converted by animal tissues into the 20-carbon vitamin A:

Vitamin A, retinol, composed of four isoprenoid units. The dotted lines indicate the junctions of the isoprenoid units.

Retinol is converted in the retina to retinal, a component of the light-sensitive pigment, rhodopsin (visual purple). A dietary deficiency of retinol may lead to night blindness, and a severe deficiency results in xerophthalmia, a blindness due to the abnormal deposition of keratin as a film over the cornea. When a person is deficient in vitamin A, the epithelial cells of all structures tend to become keratinized. The ducts of all types of glands may become blocked, leading to atrophy of the glands. Atrophy of the germinal epithelium of the testis causes sterility in the male. Skeletal growth ceases in children with vitamin A deficiency, apparently because of defective synthesis of chondroitin sulfate.

Retinoic acid can partially replace retinol in the rat diet, since it promotes the growth of bone and soft tissues, as well as the production of sperm; however, it cannot be used in the visual process. Retinoic acid is converted in experimental animals to some unknown form that is several times more active than the parent compound. The effective form of vitamin A in the body and its role in promoting the growth of bones and other tissues remain unknown. An excess of vitamin A is toxic, and acute poisoning with vitamin A has occurred after the ingestion of polar bear liver, which has a very high concentration of vitamin A. Chronic toxic reactions from prolonged overdosage with vitamin preparations are more common.

VITAMIN E

α-Tocopherol, vitamin E, contains a substituted aromatic ring and a side chain of four isoprenoid units.

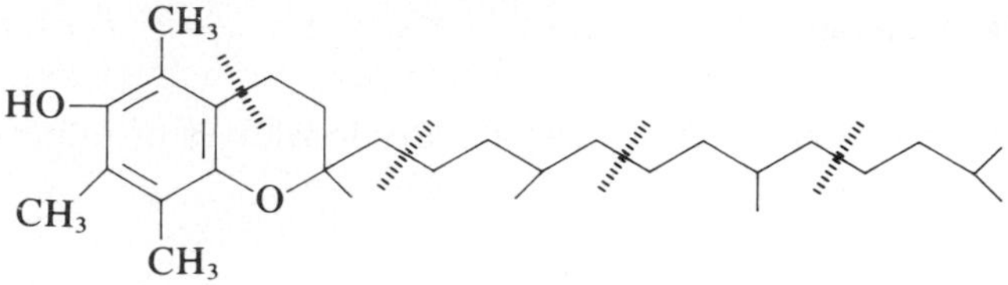

It plays some as yet unknown role in metabolism. Deficiency of vitamin E in experimental animals causes scaly skin, muscular weakness, and sterility. Tocopherol may be an antioxidant, protecting certain labile cellular components from oxidation by removing intermediate free radicals. Some investigators believe that the effects of tocopherol deficiency can be attributed to the accumulation of fatty acid peroxides, which react with and destroy other cellular components. There is some evidence that vitamin E plays a role in the mitochondrial electron transport system, but the nature of that role is unclear.

VITAMIN K

Several similar substances, referred to as vitamin K, promote the synthesis in the liver of prothrombin and proconvertin, two components of the blood-clotting mechanism. The vitamin Ks are naphthoquinones with isoprenoid side chains of varying lengths.

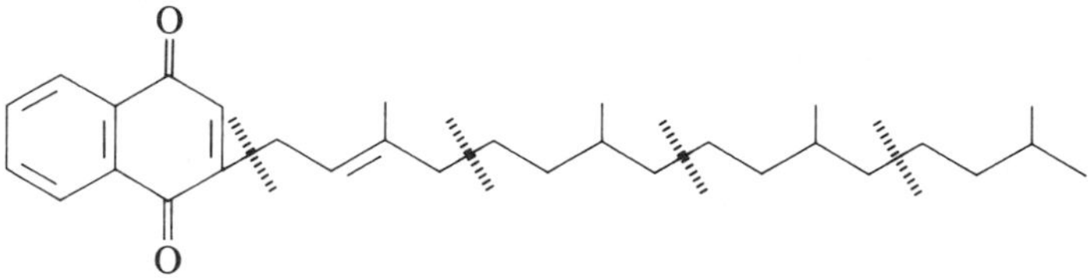

They are found in many kinds of food and are synthesized by intestinal bacteria; thus a deficiency of vitamin K is more often associated with some abnormality in its absorption than with a lack of it in the diet. Vitamin K has been shown to be a coenzyme in the carboxylation of glutamate residues in prothrombin and certain other proteins. The resulting γ-carboxyglutamate functions in binding Ca^{2+} to the protein.

Cholecalciferol: Vitamin D

Cholecalciferol leads to the mobilization of calcium and phosphate from bone and stimulates the transport of calcium across the intestinal mucosa. Cholecalciferol can be formed in the skin from 7-dehydrocholesterol by the action of ultraviolet light, which cleaves the B ring of the precursor molecule. Thus cholecalciferol is a "vitamin" only if a person is not exposed to an adequate amount of sunlight.

Cholecalciferol prevents rickets, the disease in which bones do not form properly. Rickets probably first appeared when our ancestors started wearing clothes and living in caves. By greatly reducing the amount of ultraviolet radiation of the skin, the conversion of 7α-dehydrocholesterol to cholecalciferol was reduced and, as a result, the latter compound became a vitamin, something required in the diet. At one time, rickets was prevalent in northern Europe and North America. The discovery of vitamin D in 1922 and the further discovery that sterols could be converted to vitamin D by ultraviolet irradiation made the active material readily available. Rickets has essentially been eliminated in the western world by the addition of vitamin D to milk and other foods.

One of the first clues that a metabolite of vitamin D, rather than the vitamin itself, might be the biologically active form came from the observation that there is a lag period of 10 hours or more between the administration of vitamin D and its effect on calcium transport. Two hypotheses were advanced to account for this: 1) the time might be required for the transformation of the vitamin into an active molecule, and 2) the time might be required for the synthesis of a carrier protein for calcium transport. Both of these working hypotheses have now been found to be correct. Vitamin D is converted to 25-hydroxycholecalciferol by an enzyme in the liver and then to 1,25-dihydroxycholecalciferol by an enzyme in the kidney:

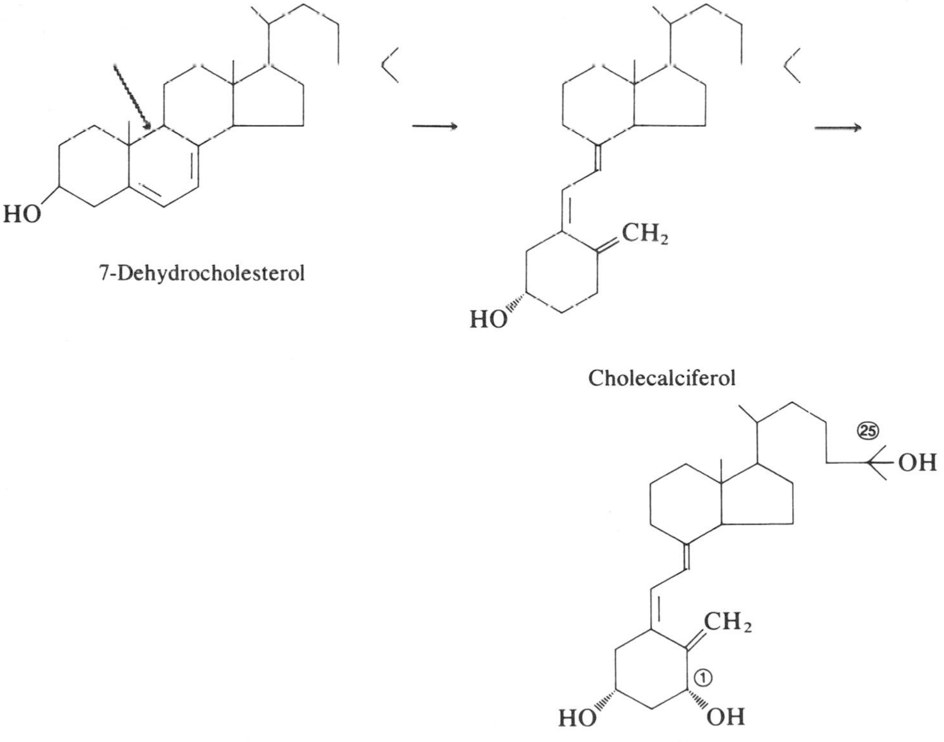

7-Dehydrocholesterol

Cholecalciferol

1,25-Dihydroxycholecalciferol

The active, hormonelike molecule (1,25-dihydroxycholecalciferol), stimulates the synthesis of a calcium transport protein in the intestinal mucosa, and this substance is responsible for the increased uptake of calcium from the intestinal contents.

Excessive doses of vitamin D are toxic, causing hypercalcemia and the deposition of calcium in soft tissues. Because it is produced in one organ (the kidney) and transported in the blood to a target tissue (the intestinal epithelial cells) where it exerts its regulatory effects, 1,25-dihydroxycholecalciferol can be considered a hormone. Its mechanism of action in the target cells closely parallels that of other steroid hormones (Fig. 4–2).

BIOSYNTHESIS OF STEROID HORMONES

Essentially the same basic pathway and the same system of enzymes is present in the adrenal gland, ovary, testis, and placenta. They result in the synthesis of five major types of steroid hormones: 1) progestins, 2) androgens, 3) estrogens, 4) glucocorticoids, and 5) mineralocorticoids. Quantitative differences and a few qualitative differences in the distribution of the steroidogenic enzymes account for the differences in the range of products of each gland. The major types of enzymes involved in steroid biosynthesis are hydroxylases, dehydrogenases, and reductases.

Cholesterol undergoes hydroxylations at positions 20α and 22. A third hydroxylation reaction leads to the cleavage of a six-carbon isocaproaldehyde fragment and leaves pregnenolone (21 carbons). The enzyme complex that catalyzes these reactions, cholesterol desmolase, is located in the mitochondria; it requires molecular oxygen, NADPH, either Mg^{2+} or Ca^{2+}, and cytochrome P_{450}.

Fig. 4–2. *Mechanism of action of steroid hormones.*

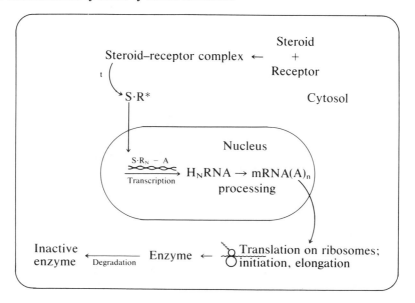

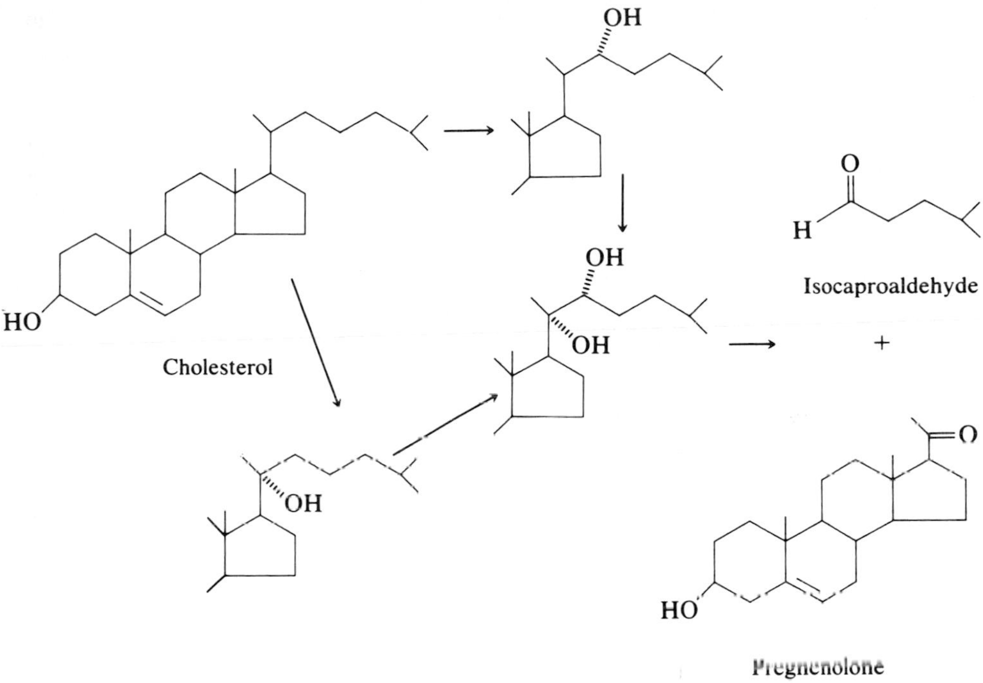

Cholesterol

Isocaproaldehyde

+

Pregnenolone

The pregnenolone formed is the major precursor of all steroid hormones and exerts a feedback regulatory influence on steroidogenesis from cholesterol by inhibiting the initial hydroxylation of the cholesterol side chain, the rate-limiting process.

A 3-β-hydroxysteroid dehydrogenase–isomerase system converts pregnenolone to progesterone. The enzyme requires NAD^+ as hydrogen acceptor and is present in the microsomal fraction.

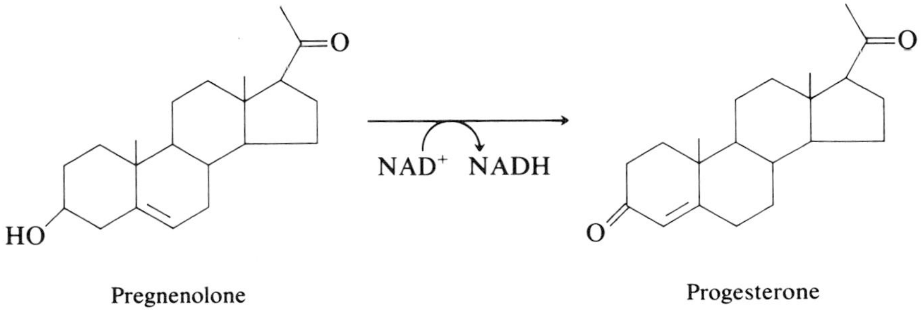

Pregnenolone

NAD^+ $NADH$

Progesterone

In the adrenal cortex, progesterone is converted to cortisol, the major glucocorticoid, and to aldosterone, the major mineralocorticoid, by a series of hydroxylation reactions (Fig. 4–3). The steroid-hydroxylating enzymes, each specific for an individual position on the steroid nucleus, are mixed function oxidases that use molecular oxygen, NADPH, adrenodoxin, and cytochrome P_{450}. In the for-

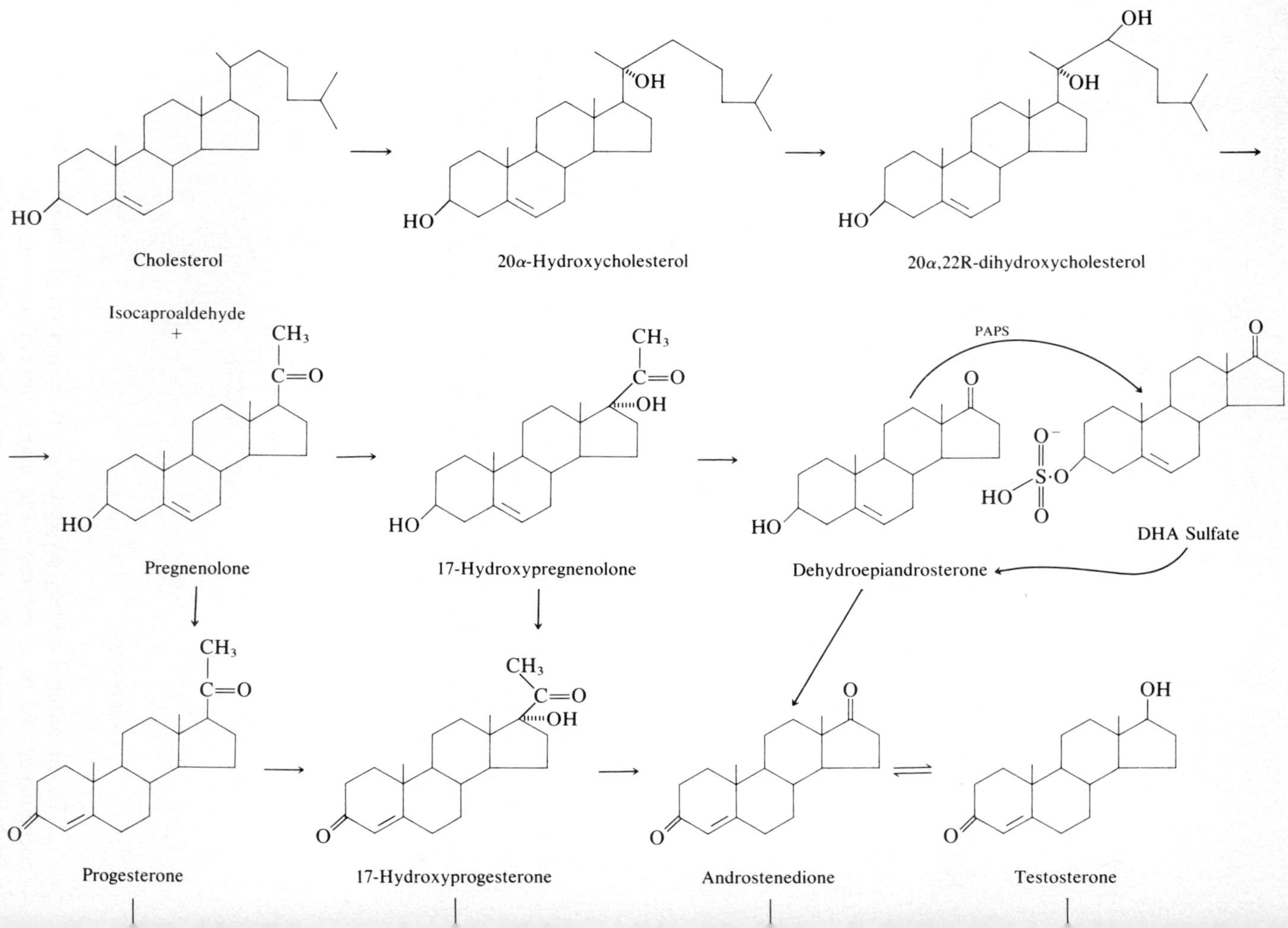

Cholesterol

20α-Hydroxycholesterol

20α,22R-dihydroxycholesterol

Isocaproaldehyde
+

17-Hydroxypregnenolone

Pregnenolone

Dehydroepiandrosterone

DHA Sulfate

PAPS

Progesterone

17-Hydroxyprogesterone

Androstenedione

Testosterone

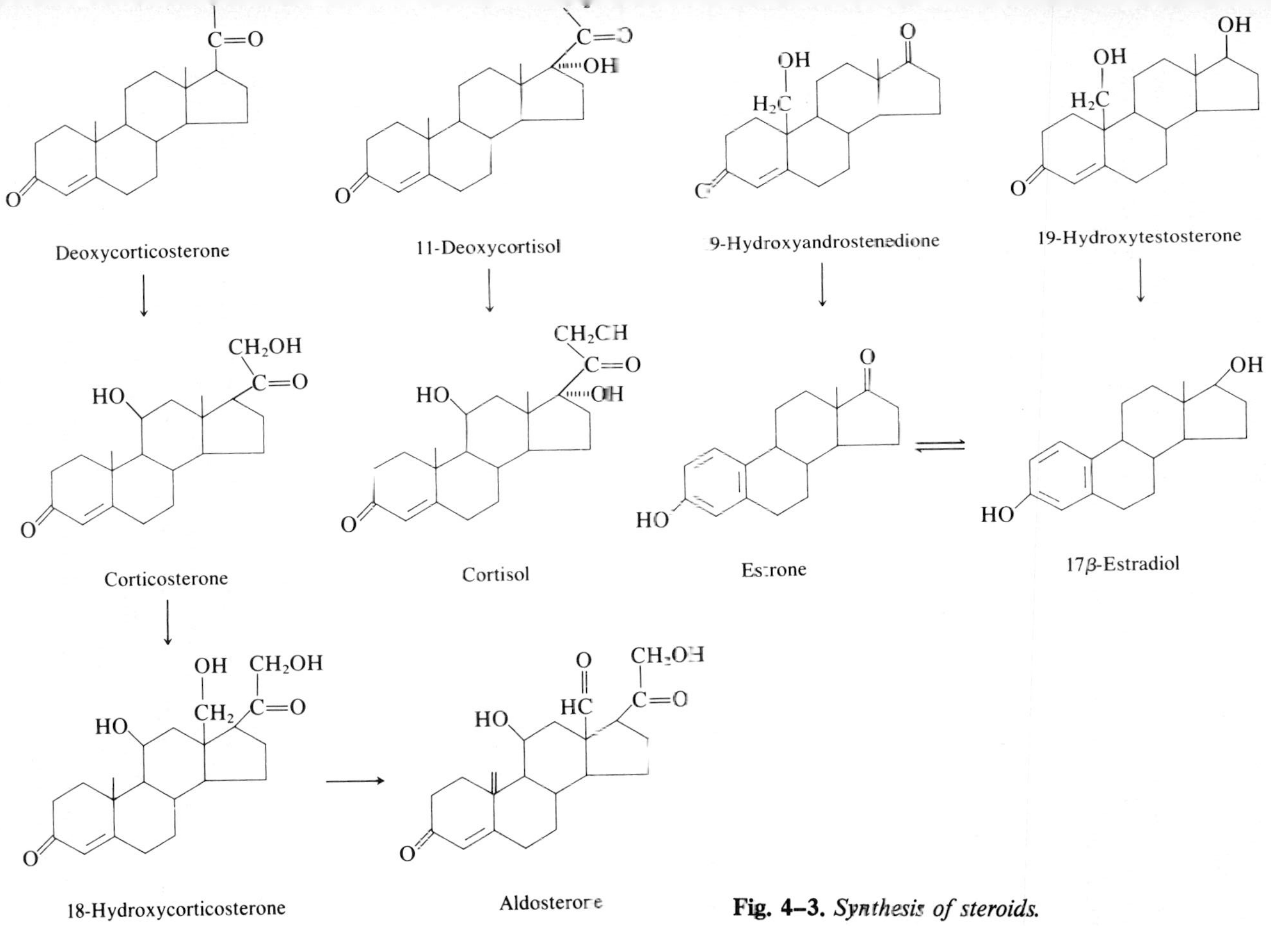

Fig. 4–3. *Synthesis of steroids.*

19-Hydroxytestosterone

17β-Estradiol

9-Hydroxyandrostenedione

Estrone

11-Deoxycortisol

Cortisol

Deoxycorticosterone

Corticosterone

18-Hydroxycorticosterone

Aldosterone

mation of cortisol, progesterone is hydroxylated at positions 17α, 21, and 11β. In the synthesis of aldosterone, progesterone is hydroxylated at positions 21, 11β, and 18 to yield 18-hydroxycorticosterone. The 18-hydroxy group is then oxidized to the aldehyde stage to yield aldosterone.

Pregnenolone undergoes 17-hydroxylation to form 17α-hydroxypregnenolone, and this can serve as substrate for the 3β-hydroxysteroid dehydrogenase–isomerase system to yield 17α-hydroxyprogesterone, which can undergo hydroxylations at positions 21 and 11β to form cortisol.

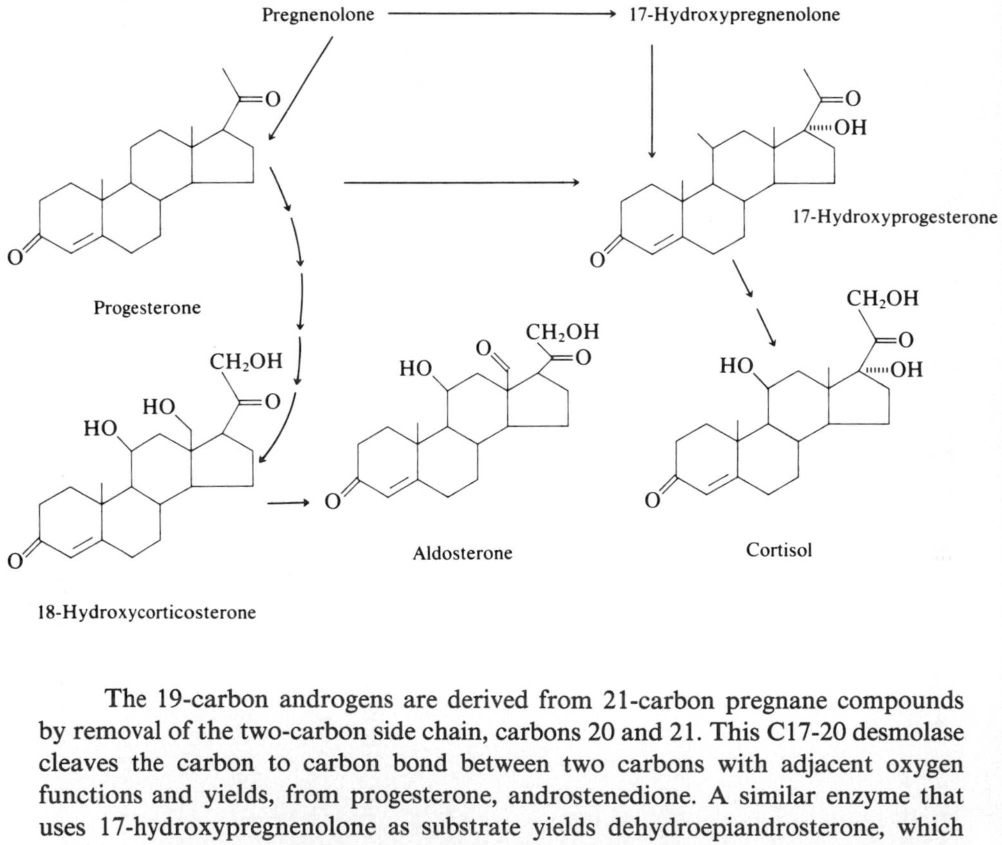

The 19-carbon androgens are derived from 21-carbon pregnane compounds by removal of the two-carbon side chain, carbons 20 and 21. This C17-20 desmolase cleaves the carbon to carbon bond between two carbons with adjacent oxygen functions and yields, from progesterone, androstenedione. A similar enzyme that uses 17-hydroxypregnenolone as substrate yields dehydroepiandrosterone, which can be converted to androstenedione by the 3β-hydroxysteroid dehydrogenase–isomerase system. Androstenedione then undergoes reduction of the oxygen function at position 17 to yield testosterone. In many tissues, the active androgen is 5α-dihydrotestosterone, derived from testosterone by reduction of the double bond between carbons 3 and 4.

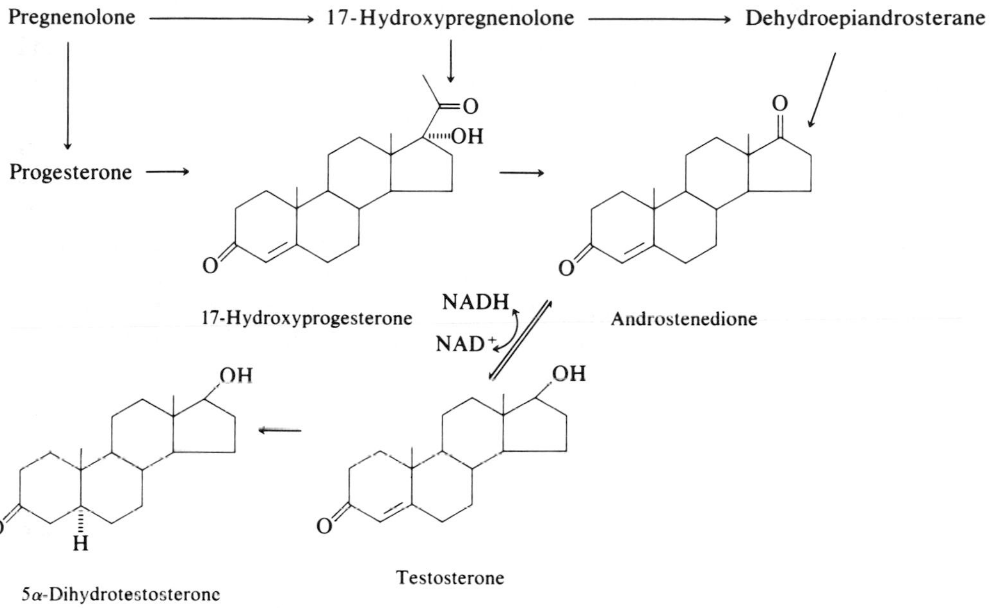

Pregnenolone ⟶ 17-Hydroxypregnenolone ⟶ Dehydroepiandrosterane

Progesterone ⟶

17-Hydroxyprogesterone

NADH
NAD⁺

Androstenedione

5α-Dihydrotestosterone

Testosterone

Estrogens are synthesized from androgens. Three hydroxylations, each requiring molecular oxygen, NADPH, and cytochrome P_{450}, carry out the conversion. The first two hydroxylations occur at the C19 methyl group, resulting in 19-hydroxytestosterone, then 19-aldehyde testosterone. The third hydroxylation occurs at carbon 2 and is the rate-determining step in the production of estrogens. The product of this last hydroxylation is rapidly and nonenzymatically converted to 17β-estradiol. This sequence of reactions, by which ring A is converted to the phenolic ring characteristic of estrogens, is termed *aromatization*.

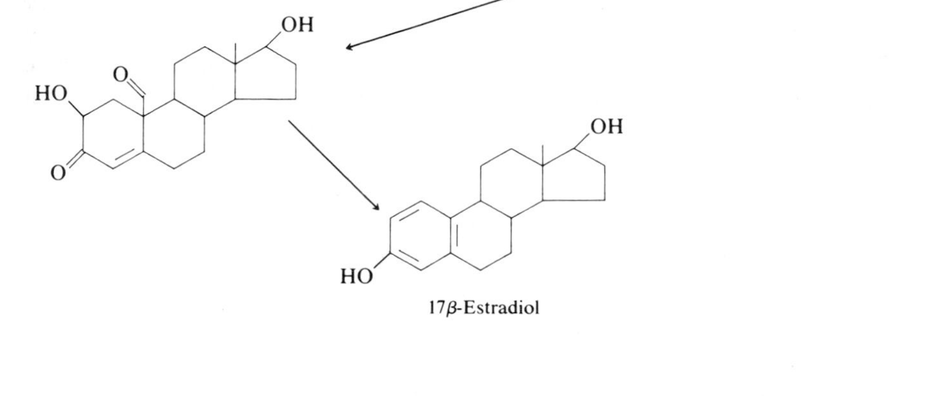

Testosterone

17β-Estradiol

Mixed Function Oxidases and Steroid Hydroxylation

The enzymes that hydroxylate steroids are mixed function oxidases that use molecular oxygen and NADPH. The overall reaction is

$$RH + O_2 + NADPH \rightarrow ROH + NADP^+ + H_2O$$

Steroid hydroxylations involve a unique electron transport system in which a cytochrome P_{450} serves as the terminal oxidase. The functional iron atom is present in the heme of an autooxidizable cytochrome; its carbon monoxide compound has an unusual absorption maximum at 450 nm. Other components of the system are a flavoprotein dehydrogenase, a nonheme iron-containing pigment (adrenodoxin), and the cytochrome P_{450}. NADPH transfers its electrons to the flavoprotein and then to adrenodoxin. This transfers an electron to the oxidized form of cytochrome P_{450}, reducing it in a reaction catalyzed by cytochrome P_{450} reductase. The reduced cytochrome P_{450} then activates oxygen.

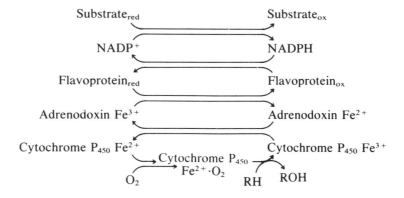

Regulation of Steroid Biosynthesis

Adrenocorticotropic hormone (ACTH) stimulates the production of steroids in the adrenal gland, and luteinizing hormone (LH) stimulates the production of steroids in the ovary or testis. The hormone-sensitive step in all steroid-producing tissues appears to be the hydroxylation of cholesterol at carbons 20 and 22 in the conversion of cholesterol to pregnenolone. ACTH and LH stimulate adenyl cyclase and the production of AMP in their respective tissues, but it is not clear whether AMP is involved in the stimulation of steroidogenesis in vivo. ACTH or LH may have a direct effect on the 20α-hydroxylase. The steroidogenic response to ACTH or LH can be blocked by cycloheximide or puromycin, inhibitors of protein synthesis. The effects of ACTH in maintaining the morphologic and functional integrity of the adrenal cortex involve both ribonucleic acid (RNA) and protein synthesis.

Congenital Adrenocortical Hyperplasia

Several disorders of steroidogenesis result in hyperplasia of the adrenal cortex. Some, but not all, are characterized by virilization of the individual. They involve a deficiency of one of the enzymes required for the biosynthesis of steroids. For example, a deficiency of 21-hydroxylase or 11-hydroxylase impairs the synthesis of cortisol from 17-hydroxyprogesterone. Since a feedback mechanism involving cortisol regulates the secretion of ACTH by the pituitary, the lack of cortisol results in an oversecretion of ACTH; the adrenal cortex is stimulated to grow (hyperplasia) and to convert precursors to steroids in greater than normal amounts. This leads to an overproduction of 17-hydroxyprogesterone. The excess 17-hydroxyprogesterone is converted to androgens, androstenedione and testosterone, which results in virilization. A deficiency of the 17-hydroxylase or of the desmolase also impairs the synthesis of cortisol and leads to an oversecretion of ACTH and to adrenal cortical hyperplasia. In the absence of 17-hydroxylation, however, neither androgens nor estrogens are formed, and no virilization results (Table 4–2).

A genetic lack of 3β-hydroxysteroid dehydrogenase prevents the formation of any 4-ene-3-one steroids and results in an accumulation of steroids with the 3β-hydroxy-5-ene configuration, pregnenolone and dehydroepiandrosterone. Infants with this deficiency fail to thrive and usually do not live for more than a few months. Dehydroepiandrosterone has some androgenic activity, but it is slight Male infants usually show only partial failure of masculinization, and female infants may have some moderate virilization at birth. The lack of 18-hydroxylase prevents the formation of aldosterone and results in salt loss, but the synthesis of androgens and estrogens occurs normally.

Treating patients with 21-hydroxylase or 11-hydroxylase deficiencies with cortisol not only provides them with the cortisol needed to regulate protein and carbohydrate metabolism, but also inhibits the secretion of ACTH by the pituitary, thus decreasing adrenal hyperplasia and the production of 17-hydroxyprogesterone and its conversion to androgens.

METABOLISM OF STEROID HORMONES

Steroid hormones are usually reduced enzymatically to decrease or eliminate their biologic activity before they are conjugated and excreted. Progesterone is reduced to pregnane-3α,20α-diol and conjugated at carbon 3 with either glucuronic acid (transferred from uridine diphosphoglucuronic acid, UDPGA) or with sulfate (transferred from 3'-phosphoadenosine-5'-phosphosulfate, PAPS). Cortisol is reduced to tetrahydrocortisol, and aldosterone is reduced to tetrahydroaldosterone; both are then conjugated at carbon 21 with glucuronic acid. Testosterone is reduced to androsterone and conjugated at carbon 3 to glucuronic acid or sulfate. Estradiol undergoes hydroxylation at carbon 2, then the methoxy derivative is formed by

Table 4-2. *Adrenocortical Hyperplasia*

Enzyme Deficient	Virilization	Steroids Secreted	Urinary 17-Ketosteroids	Salt Loss	Other Comments
21-Hydroxylase	+++++	17-OH progesterone	Elevated	Often	Most common type
18-Hydroxylase	0	Corticosterone		Yes	Rare; genitals normal in both males and females
17-Hydroxylase	0	Corticosterone and 11-deoxycorticosterone	Low	No	No sex steroids produced; ambiguous genitalia, no secondary sex characteristics in males; hypertensive
11β-Hydroxylase	++++++	11-Deoxycortisol and 11-deoxycorticosteroids	Elevated	No	Usually hypertensive
3β-Hydroxysteroid dehydrogenase	+	5-ene-3β-ol compounds	Elevated	Usually	Rare; female external genitalia in males
Desmolase	0	Cholesterol	Low	Usually	Rare; female external genitalia in males

O-methylation from *S*-adenosyl methionine. The steroid is then conjugated at carbon 3 with glucuronic acid or sulfate.

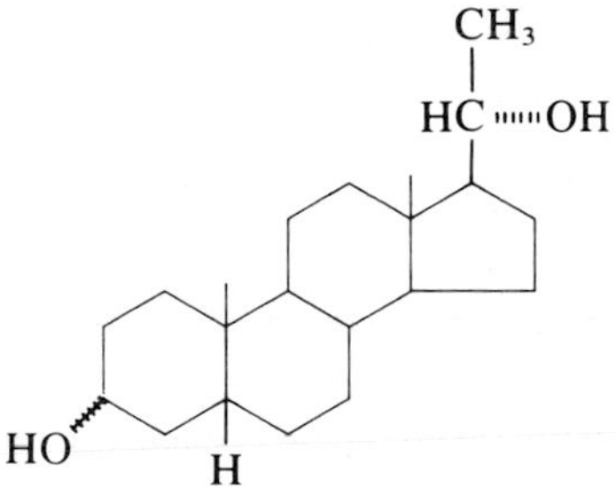

Pregnane-3α,20α-diol

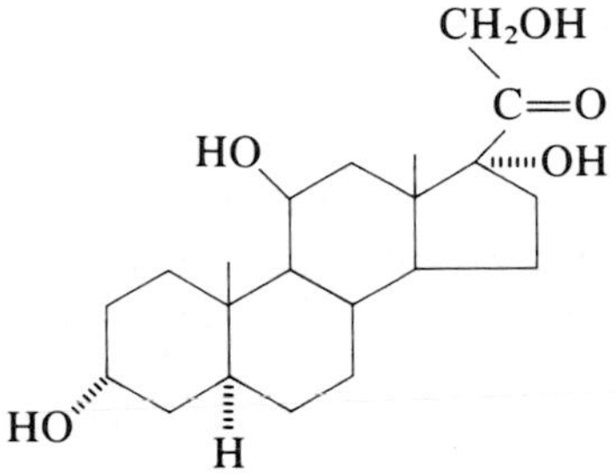

3α,5α-Tetrahydrocortisol

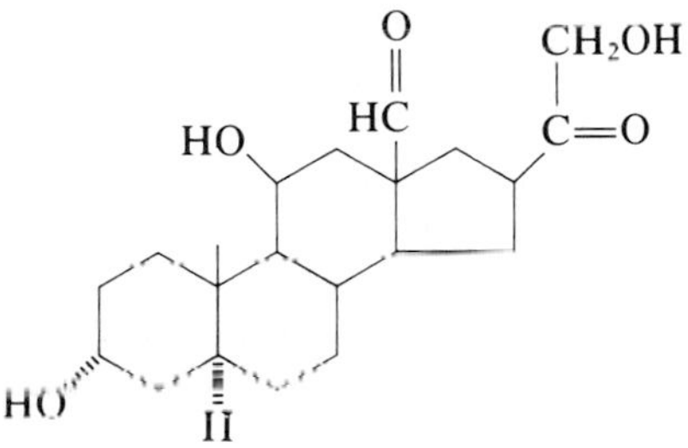

3α,5α-Tetrahydroaldosterone

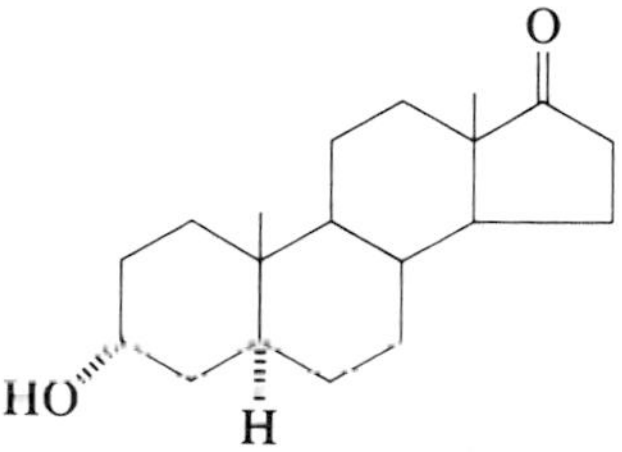

5α-Androsterone

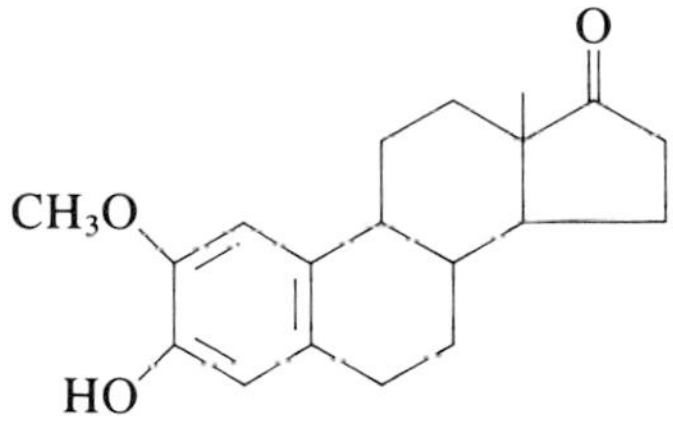

2-Methoxyestrone

STEROID HORMONES AND RECEPTORS

The synthesis of highly labeled hormones (specific activity of approximately 50 Ci/mmol) and the development of physical methods for separating specific proteins (e.g., differential density gradient ultracentrifugation, gel electrophoresis, and affinity column chromatography) made it possible to determine whether a hormone accumulates in its target tissue. In the early 1960s, Elwood Jensen demonstrated that the steroid hormone may accumulate in the target tissue without being metabolized. He postulated that target tissues have specific receptor proteins that bind the steroid, whereas those tissues that do not respond to the hormone lack these receptor proteins. Unlabeled hormone or analogs of the hormone, but not other hormones, compete for the binding sites. Autoradiography has demonstrated that labeled steroids are taken up by tissues and concentrated within the nucleus of the target cell.

Estradiol, for example, is taken up and concentrated in the uterus, vagina, mammary gland, pituitary gland, and anterior hypothalamus. Liver, kidney, muscle, and other tissues that do not respond to estradiol take up labeled estradiol, but they release it rapidly. When the uterus or other target tissue is exposed to ^{3}H-estradiol, most of the labeled hormone concentrated in the nucleus of the target tissue can be extracted by 0.4 M potassium chloride. The radioactivity is present in an estradiol–protein complex that sediments in a salt-containing sucrose gradient with a coefficient of approximately 5S. The radioactivity in the cytosol fraction sediments as an 8S steroid–protein complex when centrifuged in a low-salt sucrose gradient and as a 4S complex in a salt-containing sucrose gradient.

On entering the uterine cell, estradiol binds to a specific 4S receptor that is present in an amount greater than that needed to react with a physiologic dose of hormone. It has been estimated that there are some 100 femtomoles receptor per mg uterus in the immature rat, which corresponds to about 100,000 receptor molecules for every cell. When a dose of 0.1 μg estradiol is administered to an immature rat, the maximum amount of hormone incorporated into the uterus is about 20 femtomol per mg. The relatively unstable receptor protein is rapidly lost after the tissue is homogenized, and homogenized uterine preparations generally contain only 30 to 50 femtomol of receptor per mg uterus. The binding of the hormone to the receptor is very tight, with a dissociation constant, K_d, of about 10^{-9} M.

Several human diseases have been shown to be due to the genetic lack of a receptor. One of the most striking of these is a type of male pseudohermaphroditism termed *testicular feminization syndrome*. Individuals with this syndrome are genetic males, XY, and their testes (which may be inguinal or intraabdominal) secrete androgens at the normal male level. These individuals lack the gene that codes for the androgen receptor protein; therefore the tissues of the developing genital tract are unable to respond to the androgens, and the male sex organs cannot develop. Because, like the testes of normal males, the testes also secrete small amounts of estrogens, these individuals develop as a phenotypic female; they lack uterus or oviducts (the development of these is inhibited by Mullerian inhibiting hormone, a peptide secreted by the testis), but have a short blind pouch as a vagina. Breasts develop at puberty under the influence of estrogens, and they appear feminine. They are chromatin-negative (i.e., not XX) phenotypic females with scant pubic and axillary hair, no acne, but typically feminine proportions, voice, and habitus.

The person with diabetes insipidus excretes a large volume of urine that does not contain sugar. In the normal individual, antidiuretic hormone (ADH) produced in the hypothalamus and secreted by the posterior lobe of the pituitary gland controls the reabsorption of water from the glomerular filtrate. Diabetes insipidus results either when the hypothalamus and pituitary gland do not produce and secrete ADH or when the kidney lacks receptors for ADH. The former can be alleviated by daily injections of ADH, but the latter cannot.

MECHANISM OF ACTION OF STEROID HORMONES

The 4S estradiol–receptor complex formed in the cytosol when the estradiol initially enters the cell undergoes a temperature-dependent transformation to a 5S complex that can enter the nucleus. (The untransformed 4S complex cannot enter the nucleus.) The change from 4S to 5S appears to involve the acquisition of a second subunit. In the nucleus, the 5S estradiol–receptor complex binds to specific acceptor sites on the chromatin, leading to increased production of the messenger RNAs that code for specific proteins involved in the growth response.

The most clearly understood estrogen response is the production of ovalbumin in the chick oviduct in response to estradiol. The messenger RNA for ovalbumin has been isolated, the corresponding copy DNA (cDNA) has been synthesized by reverse transcriptase, and the gene for ovalbumin has been analyzed. It appears that steroid hormones regulate metabolism in their target cells primarily by affecting the genetic apparatus and increasing the synthesis of specific messenger RNAs and, hence, the synthesis of specific proteins. The hormonal effect can be inhibited by actinomycin D, which inhibits RNA synthesis, or by cycloheximide, which inhibits protein synthesis. Isolated nuclei of uterine cells show an increased rate of RNA synthesis when incubated with estradiol and with uterine cytosol that contains receptors.

An estrogen receptor is present in normal mammary tissue. When mammary cancer first develops, the neoplastic tissue contains the receptor and responds to estradiol; it is a hormone-dependent tumor. The receptor usually disappears with time, however, and the growth of the tumor becomes independent of hormone. Because the type of treatment used for hormone-dependent tumors differs from that used for hormone-independent tumors, biopsy specimens of mammary tumors are analyzed for the presence or absence of estrogen receptors as a clue to optimal treatment.

Comparable receptors have been found in other tissues, each specific for one class of steroids—androgens, progestins, glucocorticoids, or mineralocorticoids. Each of these has a specific sedimentation constant that differs from those of the other receptors; each is a distinctive protein. All of them are characterized by 1) high specificity (for a single kind of hormone), 2) high affinity for that specific steroid (with dissociation constants of about $10^{-9}M$), and 3) low capacity (saturable by relatively low concentrations of hormone).

Receptors for protein hormones are also highly specific, have high affinity constants, and are saturable. The receptors for protein hormones, however, are typically located in the plasma membrane of the cell rather than in the cytosol. Some protein hormone–receptor complexes appear to remain on the cell surface and produce their effects by stimulating adenyl cyclase to produce the "second messenger," AMP, which activates specific protein kinases. Other protein hormone–receptor complexes are internalized and have effects, directly or indirectly, on the genetic mechanism that parallel those of the steroid hormones.

PROSTAGLANDINS, THROMBOXANES, AND LEUKOTRIENES

Prostaglandins and thromboxanes are polyunsaturated, hydroxylated, long-chain fatty acids with remarkable biologic activities at extremely low concentrations. Their discovery was due largely to the efforts of a single group working under Ulf von Euler at the Karolinska Institute in Stockholm. Von Euler showed in the early 1930s that extracts of semen or of the prostate gland can be used to decrease blood pressure and to stimulate contractions in strips of smooth muscle isolated from the uterus or intestine. In 1960, Sune Bergstrom isolated the first two prostaglandins. When partitioned between ether and aqueous phosphate buffer the one more soluble in ether was called prostaglandin E (ether) and the one more soluble in phosphate buffer was called prostaglandin F (Swedish *fosfat*). When minced sheep vesicular gland is incubated at 37°, the prostaglandin content increases tenfold within a few minutes, indicating that prostaglandin is being actively synthesized. It is now known that the prostaglandins in human semen are synthesized primarily by the seminal vesicle rather than by the prostate. Despite the incorrect original assumption which gave rise to the name "prostaglandin" it has not been changed.

Prostaglandins are synthesized by and function in virtually all organs of the body. The chemical names of all the prostaglandins and their metabolites are derived by reference to the 20-carbon prostanoic acid:

Prostanoic acid

Members of all four naturally occurring series of prostaglandins (i.e., E, F, A, and B) are hydroxylated at carbon 15 and have a trans double bond between carbons 13 and 14. The number of double bonds is indicated by the subscript numeral after the letter. Thus, prostaglandin E_1 and F_1 have a single trans double bond between carbons 13 and 14. Prostaglandins E_2 and F_2 have an additional cis double bond between carbons 5 and 6. Prostaglandins in the F series have an hydroxyl group rather than a ketone group at position 9. Thus, there are two isomeric alcohols, F_α with the OH group below the plane of the cyclopentane ring and F_β with the hydroxyl group above the cyclopentane ring. All of the naturally occurring prostaglandins F are F_α.

Thromboxane and prostacyclin are potent cellular regulatory agents. Derived from the same precursors as prostaglandins, they are involved in the regulation of platelet aggregation.

Biosynthesis of Prostaglandins

Arachidonic acid, which has 20 carbons and four double bonds, is synthesized from linoleic acid, which has 18 carbons and two double bonds, by an elongation reaction using malonyl CoA and by two desaturation reactions that involve the removal of hydrogens and the introduction of double bonds. Arachidonic acid may be abbreviated as $5,8,11,14\text{-}C_{20:4}$. The prefix numbers indicate the location of the double bonds, the subscript indicates the total number of carbon atoms, and the number after the colon indicates the total number of double bonds. Much of the arachidonic acid in a tissue is esterified to the glycerol of phospholipids and is present in the lipid bilayer of membranes. The first step in the synthesis of prostaglandins is the release of arachidonic acid from membrane phospholipids in a reaction catalyzed by phospholipase A_2.

The conversion of arachidonic acid to prostaglandin is catalyzed by prostaglandin synthetase, also termed prostaglandin cyclooxygenase. This enzyme has been highly purified from the microsomal fraction of sheep vesicular glands and has been shown to contain nonheme iron, as well as loosely bound heme. The addition of glutathione or hydroquinone, which serve as antioxidants, increases the yield of prostaglandin, but the addition of ATP or NADH does not. Many kinds of prostaglandins and prostaglandinlike compounds are produced when eicosatrienoic ($C_{20:3}$) or eicosatetraenoic acid (arachidonic, $C_{20:4}$) are incubated with the microsomal sheep vesicular gland preparation. Samuelson showed that the oxygen atoms, added at positions 9, 11, and 15 are derived from molecular oxygen and that the oxygen atom at carbon 9 is derived from the same molecule of oxygen as the oxygen atom at carbon 11. From these and other experiments, Samuelson and his colleagues proposed that the first intermediate in the biosynthesis of prostaglandins is an 11-peroxy-8,12,14 eicosatrienoic acid and that this is cyclized into an endoperoxide (Fig. 4–4).

The first step in the sequence of reactions catalyzed by the cyclooxygenase is the elimination of a hydrogen ion from carbon 13, leaving a free radical. Thereafter the addition of the peroxy radical to positions 9 and 11, the formation of the 8,12 carbon–carbon bond subsequent to the isomerization of the 11,12 double bond to a 12,13 double bond, and the addition of another peroxy radical at position 15 (resulting in the isomerization of the 12,13 double bond to the 13,14 double bond) are envisioned as proceeding by one electron shifts. The first product of this reaction is 15-hydroperoxy-9,11-endoperoxide, prostaglandin G_2. The endoperoxides, prostaglandins G_1 and H_1, are transformed to prostaglandins E_1 and $F_{1\alpha}$. Beginning with arachidonic acid (eicosatetraenoic acid), the resulting prostaglandins G_2 and H_2 are converted to prostaglandins E_2 and $F_{2\alpha}$. These endoperoxide intermediates

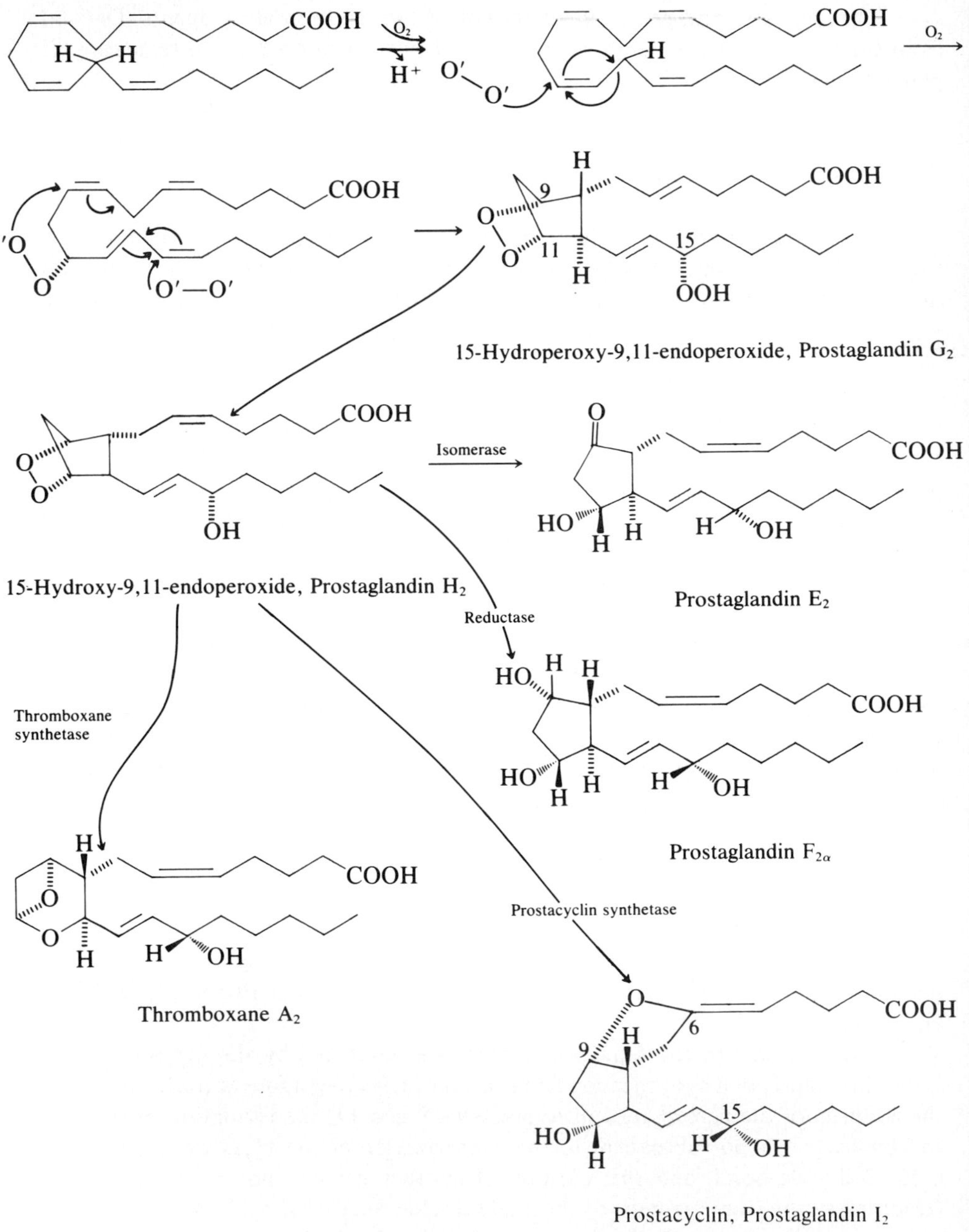

15-Hydroperoxy-9,11-endoperoxide, Prostaglandin G_2

15-Hydroxy-9,11-endoperoxide, Prostaglandin H_2

Isomerase

Prostaglandin E_2

Reductase

Prostaglandin $F_{2\alpha}$

Thromboxane synthetase

Thromboxane A_2

Prostacyclin synthetase

Prostacyclin, Prostaglandin I_2

Fig. 4–4. *Biosynthesis of prostaglandins and thromboxanes from arachidonic acid.*

are unstable in aqueous media and have very short half-lives. The prostaglandin endoperoxides inhibit hormone-stimulated cAMP accumulation in platelets and adipocytes, which may be the mechanism by which the endoperoxides induce the aggregation of platelets. The endoperoxide prostaglandin H_2 is converted to prostaglandin E_2 by an isomerase and to prostaglandin $F_{2\alpha}$ by a reductase (Fig. 4–4).

Arachidonic acid can be hydroxylated at carbon 12, yielding 12-hydroxyeicosatetraenoic acid, by the enzyme lipoxygenase. This substance, one of the leukotrienes, has potent chemotactic activity in cultured cells.

Samuelson and his colleagues estimated the production rate of prostaglandin E by measuring the amount of urinary metabolites. In adult males, the production rate ranged from 109 to 226 $\mu g/24$ hours. In adult females, it ranged from 23 to 48 $\mu g/24$ hours. These results suggest that there is a sex difference in the production of prostagandins and that only a small fraction of the precursor essential fatty acids consumed in the diet are converted to prostaglandins. The amount of linoleic acid consumed in the diet is on the order of 10 $g/24$ hours.

Platelets, the spleen, and the lung contain a thromboxane synthetase that produces thromboxane from prostaglandin H_2. Thromboxanes contain a six-membered ring with five carbons and an oxygen atom; the second oxygen is present as an epoxide joining carbons 9 and 11.

The lining of blood vessels contains an enzyme, prostacyclin synthetase, that converts the endoperoxide prostaglandin H_2 to prostacyclin, which has an epoxide bridge between carbons 6 and 9.

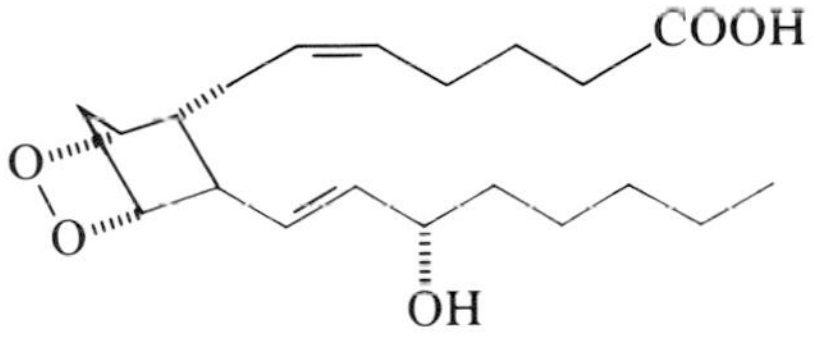

15-Hydroxy-9,11-endoperoxide, Prostaglandin H_2

Prostacyclin synthetase

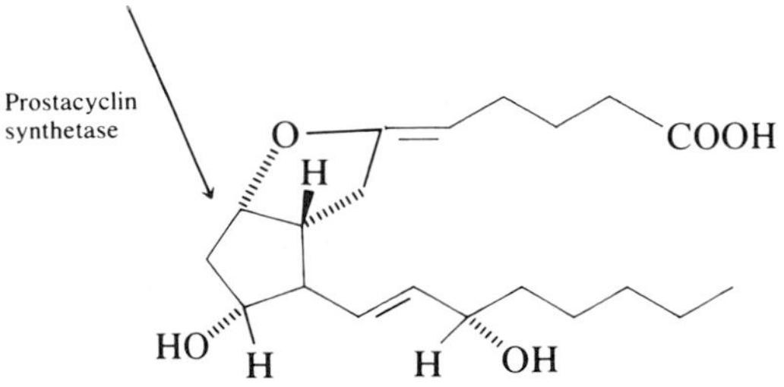

Prostacyclin, Prostaglandin I_2

The prostaglandin cyclooxygenase is under an unusual type of control. The initial oxidation catalyzed by the enzyme proceeds for a brief period and then stops, apparently because of a self-catalyzed destruction of the cyclooxygenase.

This type of control permits a finite, limited response that does not depend on the diffusion of some distant product back to a regulatory site to halt enzyme activity, as is typically the case with soluble cytoplasmic feedback systems. This limiting property of the enzyme necessitates new protein synthesis to increase enzyme activity and, therefore, the selective induction of messenger RNA coding for that enzyme. Thus, the variety of hormones and hormone-regulated interactions that influence the synthesis of messenger RNA and protein can determine the length of time that a tissue cannot synthesize additional prostaglandins.

As part of their pharmacologic action, many common drugs appear to modify the synthesis of prostaglandins. Prostaglandins are potent inflammatory agents. Aspirin and nonsteroid, antiinflammatory drugs, such as indomethacin, reduce inflammation by inhibiting prostaglandin cyclooxygenase. It is postulated that aspirin donates an acetyl group to the enzyme, which inactivates it. Glucocorticoids also have an antiinflammatory action; they inhibit phospholipase A_2, which releases the precursor, arachidonic acid, from its bound form in the phospholipid of the membrane. This decreases the rate of prostaglandin synthesis.

The K_m of prostacyclin synthetase for the endoperoxide appears to be lower than those of the enzymes involved in the synthesis of prostaglandins. If the system contains only a small amount of arachidonic acid, the product is largely prostacyclin. With higher levels of arachidonic acid, the major products are the prostaglandins E_2 and $F_{2\alpha}$. Prostacyclin synthetase is present in cells other than endothelial cells, such as the brain and the corpus luteum.

The natural prostaglandins, thromboxanes, and prostacyclins all have very short biologic half-lives. An intensive search has been made for a synthetic prostaglandin analog that would have a much longer half-life and could be used clinically. 15-Methyl prostaglandin $F_{2\alpha}$ appears promising. In the degradation of prostaglandins, the conversion of the 15-hydroxy group to a 15-keto group results in almost complete loss of biologic activities. The presence of the methyl group prevents this conversion and greatly lengthens the biologic half-life of the prostaglandin.

Metabolism of Prostaglandins

Prostaglandins are converted to a number of metabolites and excreted in the urine. In most of these, the carbon chain has been shortened by two or four carbons. Dinor prostaglandin lacks two carbons, and tetranor prostaglandin lacks four carbons. The oxidation of the secondary alcohol at carbon 15 to a ketonic function, and the reduction of the trans double bond between carbons 13 and 14 occur in reactions catalyzed by enzymes present in the lung. The shortening of the carboxyl side chain by β-oxidation probably occurs in the liver.

Some 95% of prostaglandin is removed in one circulation through the lung, and 80% of prostaglandin infused into the hepatic portal vein is removed as it passes through the liver. These processes account for the very short half-life of the

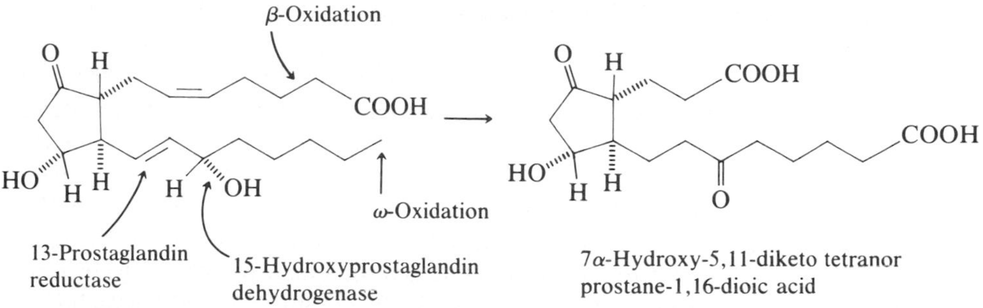

β-Oxidation

13-Prostaglandin reductase

15-Hydroxyprostaglandin dehydrogenase

ω-Oxidation

7α-Hydroxy-5,11-diketo tetranor prostane-1,16-dioic acid

prostaglandins. The body has efficient mechanisms for preventing prostaglandins from reaching the arterial circulation and decreasing arterial pressure.

Prostaglandin dehydrogenase, which converts prostaglandins to the 15-oxo derivatives, requires NAD as hydrogen acceptor. A second 15-hydroxy prostaglandin dehydrogenase that uses NADP as hydrogen acceptor has been found in the brain, erythrocytes, and kidney. Prostaglandin reductase, which reduces the $C_{13,14}$ double bond, is present in the particle-free fraction of many tissues and uses $FADH_2$ as the hydrogen donor. Prostaglandins also serve as substrates for the fatty acid β-oxidation system in rat liver mitochondria. The carboxyl side chain is degraded by the removal of 1 or 2 two-carbon fragments. The prostaglandin chain may also undergo ω-oxidation, yielding compounds with a carboxyl group at carbon 20. This may then undergo β-oxidation, and the chain can be shortened at both the α and ω ends.

Thromboxane A_2 is rapidly converted to the inactive thromboxane B_2 by an enzyme catalyzed cleavage of the epoxy bridge between carbons 9 and 11, and their reduction to hydroxyl groups. Prostacyclin is converted to 6-keto-$PGF_{1\alpha}$ and excreted.

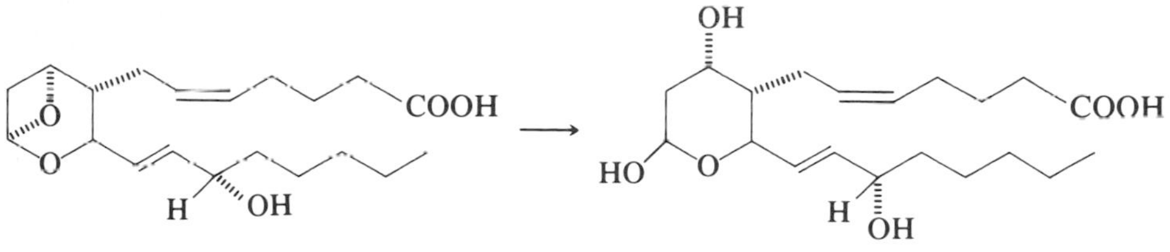

Thromboxane A_2

Thromboxane B_2

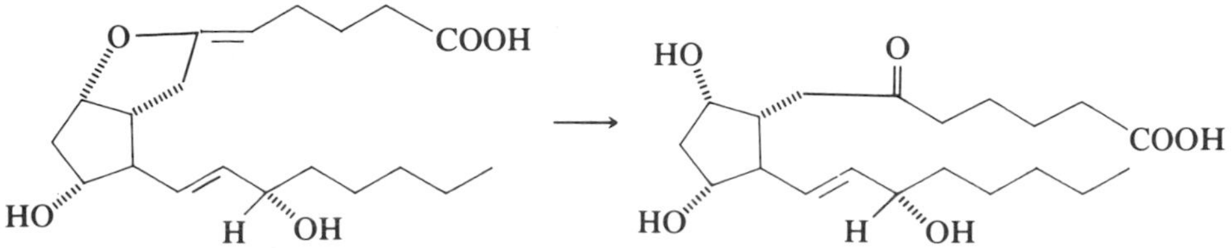

Prostacyclin

6-Keto-$PGF_{1\alpha}$

Physiologic Roles of Prostaglandins

The myometrium of the pregnant woman is especially sensitive to the prostaglandins $F_{2\alpha}$ and E_2. The fact that the myometrium responds to these prostaglandins by contracting is the basis for their use as agents to increase uterine contractions during parturition and for their use as abortifacients. Prostaglandins have a variety of effects on blood vessels and on the cardiovascular system. The specific effects depend on the kind of prostaglandin used and the species of animal. Prostaglandins E_1, E_2, and A reduce systemic arterial blood pressure. The infusion of prostaglandin E_1 not only causes tachycardia, facial flushing, and headache, but also decreases cardiac output and systemic arterial blood pressure. Prostaglandin $F_{2\alpha}$, widely used as an abortifacient, has no effect on systolic or diastolic blood pressure or on heart or respiratory rate. Prostaglandins decrease the secretion of acid and pepsin by gastric mucosa, as well as the total volume of gastric juice. Their side effects include massive reflux of bile into the stomach and greatly increased intestinal motility, resulting in vomiting and diarrhea, however.

Blood platelets produce thromboxane A_2, which causes marked aggregation of platelets and constriction of vascular smooth muscle. The cells in the endothelial walls produce prostacyclin, the effects of which oppose those of thromboxane. When endothelial cells are intact, the prostacyclin produced by the endothelium prevents platelet aggregation. When the vascular wall is damaged, platelets tend to aggregate in that area because of the local depressed concentration of prostacyclin.

Karim suggested in 1969 that prostaglandins may play a physiologic role in inducing uterine contractions at parturition, and showed that they could be used successfully to induce labor. The intravenous administration of prostaglandin $F_{2\alpha}$ induces abortion in early pregnancy by stimulating uterine activity so that fetus and placenta are expelled. The marked side effects of nausea and diarrhea associated with intravenous administration can be minimized by administering the prostaglandin intravaginally or into the uterine cavity, and by administering 15-methyl prostaglandins.

5

Metabolism of Nitrogenous Compounds

Digestion of Proteins and Uptake of Amino Acids
Cofactors
Essential Amino Acids
Deamination
Transamination
Glutamic Dehydrogenase
Ammonia and Its Metabolism
Carbamoyl Phosphate
Urea Cycle
Inherited Enzyme Deficiencies
Hyperammonemia
Citrullinemia
Argininosuccinic Acidemia
Metabolism of Methionine and Cysteine
Cystinuria
Cystinosis
Branched Chain Amino Acids
Metabolism of Valine, Leucine, and Isoleucine
Maple Syrup Urine Disease
Isovaleric Acidemia and Jamaican Vomiting
Disease
Heterocyclic Amino Acids
Metabolism of Tryptophan
Metabolism of Histidine
Metabolism of Phenylalanine and Tyrosine
Production of Catecholamines
Melanin and Albinism
Biosynthesis of Thyroxine

The oxidation of carbohydrates and lipids supplies most, up to 90%, of the energy requirements of the adult human. Although it is obvious that the carbon chains of the amino acids can be fed into the glycolytic or tricarboxylic acid cycles and undergo reactions that will produce biologically useful energy, intracellular amino acids serve primarily as substrates for the synthesis of proteins. They can lose their amino groups by transamination or deamination, and the resulting α-keto acids undergo oxidation to carbon dioxide and water. In addition, amino acids serve as precursors of several nitrogen-containing compounds of physiologic importance, such as creatine, purines, pyrimidines, porphyrins, and polyamines. The amino groups removed in transamination or deamination are excreted as ammonia, urea, or uric acid.

Many diseases are caused by inherited deficiencies of one or another of the enzymes involved in the metabolism of amino acids. These inborn errors of metabolism, caused by the lack of the gene that codes for the enzyme, may lead to the accumulation of some toxic intermediate or prevent the formation of a product that is required for health. The loss of some control system that regulates the overall pathway may also result in disease.

Neither proteins nor free amino acids are "stored" within a cell as glycogen and triacylglycerols are. The proteins in a cell are all functional, either as enzymes or as structural components of the cytoplasm. The pool of free amino acids in a cell is small and consists of the immediate precursors of proteins and the other complex, nitrogen-containing compounds. Unlike glucose and fatty acids, amino acids do not generally require activation with adenosine triphosphate (ATP) to undergo metabolism. In some reactions, however, amino acids do react with ATP and transfer ribonucleic acid to form the substrates for the synthesis of peptide chains. The metabolism of nitrogen-containing compounds is illustrated in Figure 5–1.

DIGESTION OF PROTEINS AND UPTAKE OF AMINO ACIDS

Proteins in food are digested by proteolytic enzymes in the stomach and intestine. The resulting amino acids are rapidly taken up into the bloodstream by

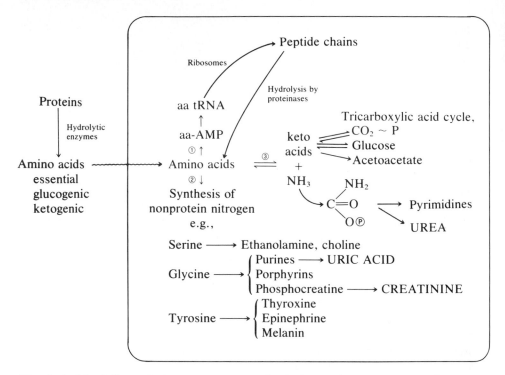

Fig. 5–1. *Metabolism of nitrogenous compounds: Amino acids, purines, pyrimidines, porphyrins, melanin, catecholamines, creatinine phosphate, and peptides.*

active, energy-requiring processes. There appear to be at least five specific transport systems for amino acids, each for a different group of closely similar amino acids. The uptake of any amino acid is inhibited by an excess of any of the other amino acids in the same group. Similar transport systems function in the uptake of amino acids from the plasma by the liver, skeletal muscle, and other cells. The uptake of amino acids from the plasma is rapid—some 85% or more of an injected 5- to 10-g dose is removed from the plasma within 5 minutes.

Within the cell, the amino acid has three possible fates. First, it may be activated by ATP to the amino acid adenylate and transferred to transfer RNA to be incorporated into a nascent peptide chain on the ribosome. Peptide chains may undergo hydrolysis within the cell by proteinases in the lysosomes, and the resulting amino acids are returned to the intracellular amino acid pool. Second, certain amino acids are involved in the synthesis of specific "nonprotein nitrogen" compounds. Serine and its metabolic products, ethanolamine and choline, are constituents of phospholipids, such as phosphatidyl choline. The smallest amino acid, glycine, has an important role in the biosynthesis of purines, porphyrins, and phosphocreatine. Tyrosine is a precursor of the hormones thyroxine and epinephrine, and of the black pigment melanin. Third, after the removal of the amino group, the carbon chain of the corresponding α-keto acid may be metabolized in the tricarboxylic acid cycle with the generation of energy-rich phosphate groups, or it may be converted to glucose or to acetoacetate and the other ketone bodies.

COFACTORS

Just as nicotinamide adenine dinucleotide (NAD) and flavin adenine dinucleotide (FAD) are the typical cofactors of dehydrogenations, and thiamine pyrophosphate and lipoic acid are the typical cofactors of the oxidative decarboxylation of keto acids, pyridoxal phosphate is a cofactor in most of the reactions of amino acids, such as transamination and decarboxylation. Folic acid and its derivatives are involved in the metabolism and interconversion of one-carbon compounds derived from amino acids and used in the biosynthesis of purines.

ESSENTIAL AMINO ACIDS

Like the essential fatty acids, the essential amino acids cannot be synthesized by human cells and must be contained in the diet. Human cells lack certain enzymes present in plants that catalyze the synthesis of the corresponding α-keto acid. If presented with the corresponding α-keto acid in the diet, however, the human can convert it into the essential amino acid. The amino acids essential for growth in the human include leucine, isoleucine, valine, lysine, tryptophan, phenylalanine, methionine, and threonine. Tyrosine is not an essential amino acid, for humans can synthesize it from phenylalanine present in the diet.

A 70-kg man synthesizes and degrades some 400 g protein per day. His diet provides about 160 g protein, and the pancreatic enzymes that are synthesized and secreted account for as much as 100 g protein per day. There is very little free amino acid in the urine. In an adult, there is no net increase in the protein content of the body over long periods of time; an amount of amino acid equivalent to that ingested must undergo degradation. It is remarkable that in the adult the rates of synthesis and degradation are so neatly balanced.

Those amino acids with a carbon chain (or a portion of it) that can be converted to glucose are glucogenic amino acids. Gluconeogenesis refers to the synthesis of new glucose chains from noncarbohydrate precursors, primarily from amino acids. The carbon chain of the amino acid is converted by a series of intermediates to phosphoenol pyruvate and the carbons of phosphoenolpyruvate are converted to glucose by a reversal of glycolysis. Alanine, aspartate, glutamate, and serine are glucogenic amino acids. Those amino acids with a carbon chain (or some portion of it) that can be converted to acetyl CoA and thus to acetoacetate, β-hydroxybutyrate, and acetone are ketogenic amino acids. Phenylalanine, tyrosine, lysine, and isoleucine are amino acids that are in part glucogenic and in part ketogenic. Leucine is ketogenic only.

Amino groups are removed from amino acids by oxidative deamination, by transamination, or by glutamic dehydrogenase. Amino acids can be synthesized from the corresponding α-keto acid by the reverse process.

Deamination

The oxidative deamination of amino acids occurs primarily in the liver and, to a smaller extent, in the kidney. A hepatectomized animal has a greatly reduced ability to remove amino acids from the blood and to synthesize urea. The liver and kidney contain enzymes that can liberate ammonia from amino acids by oxidative processes in which 2 mol ammonia are formed for each mol oxygen taken up. In addition to the enzymes that oxidize the naturally occurring L-α-amino acids, a spectrum of D-amino acid oxidases use as substrates the D-amino acids not usually found as constituents of peptides. Both D- and L-amino acid oxidases are flavoproteins.

$$
\underset{\underset{NH_2}{|}}{R-CH-CO_2H} + FP \longrightarrow \left[\underset{NH}{\overset{\parallel}{R \cdot C \cdot CO_2H}} \right] + H_2FP
$$

$$
+ H_2O \searrow \quad \underset{O}{\overset{\parallel}{R \cdot C \cdot CO_2H}} + NH_3
$$

Transamination

Amino groups are transferred from one amino acid to another by way of reactions catalyzed by aminotransferases that use pyridoxal phosphate as coenzyme. In essence, the amino group is first transferred to pyridoxal phosphate bound to the enzyme, converting it into pyridoxamine phosphate (still bound to the enzyme), and the pyridoxamine phosphate donates its amino group to a second keto acid, converting it to an amino acid and regenerating pyridoxal phosphate bound to the enzyme. This is then ready to attack the next amino acid. Glutamate and its α-keto acid, α-ketoglutarate, are typically one pair of reacting partners:

$$\text{Alanine} + \alpha\text{-Ketoglutarate} \rightleftarrows \text{Pyruvate} + \text{Glutamate}$$

The C=O group of the enzyme-bound pyridoxal phosphate condenses with the amino group of the amino acid to form a type of Schiff base. The C=N double bond shifts, and the carbon skeleton of the amino acid is released as an α-keto acid, with the amino group remaining bound as pyridoxamine phosphate. This then forms a Schiff base with a new α-ketoglutarate, to which the amino group is transferred by a reversal of the reactions by which it was formed. The amino transferases are named by the pair of amino acids involved (e.g., glutamate–aspartate aminotransferase).

Glutamic Dehydrogenase

A specific glutamic acid dehydrogenase, widely distributed in tissues, catalyzes the deamination of glutamic acid. It uses NAD as its cofactor. The reaction is readily reversible; in the reverse direction, it allows ammonia to be taken up by α-ketoglutarate to form glutamic acid. The amino group of glutamate may then be transferred to other amino acids by transamination. The combination of glutamic dehydrogenase and the transamination reaction provides a mechanism by which ammonia can be incorporated into the amino group of essentially any amino acid.

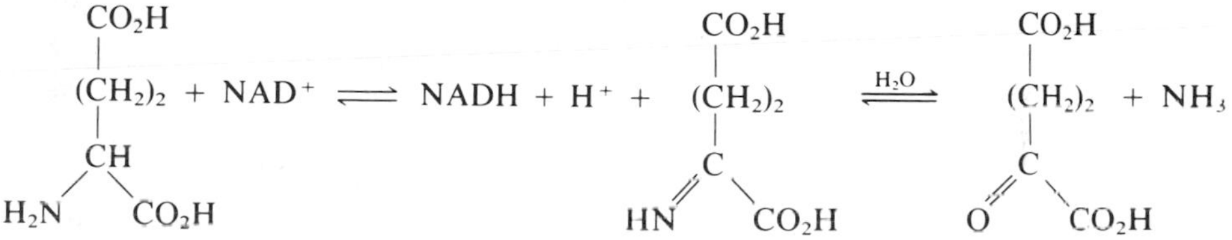

$$\begin{array}{c} CO_2H \\ | \\ (CH_2)_2 \\ | \\ CH \\ H_2N \quad CO_2H \end{array} + NAD^+ \rightleftharpoons NADH + H^+ + \begin{array}{c} CO_2H \\ | \\ (CH_2)_2 \\ | \\ C \\ HN \quad CO_2H \end{array} \xrightarrow{\text{H}_2\text{O}} \begin{array}{c} CO_2H \\ | \\ (CH_2)_2 \\ | \\ C \\ O \quad CO_2H \end{array} + NH_3$$

AMMONIA AND ITS METABOLISM

Ammonia is normally present at very low concentrations, about 2×10^{-5}M, in tissues and blood. An adult human synthesizes nearly 1 mol ammonia per day, however, partly by enzymes in the liver and partly by the bacteria in the gut. Ammonia is very toxic and is taken up primarily by glutamic dehydrogenase in the reaction with α-ketoglutarate to form glutamate (Fig. 5–2). In another reaction, catalyzed by glutamine synthetase, ammonia and ATP react with glutamate to form glutamine, adenosine diphosphate (ADP), and inorganic phosphate. Gluta-

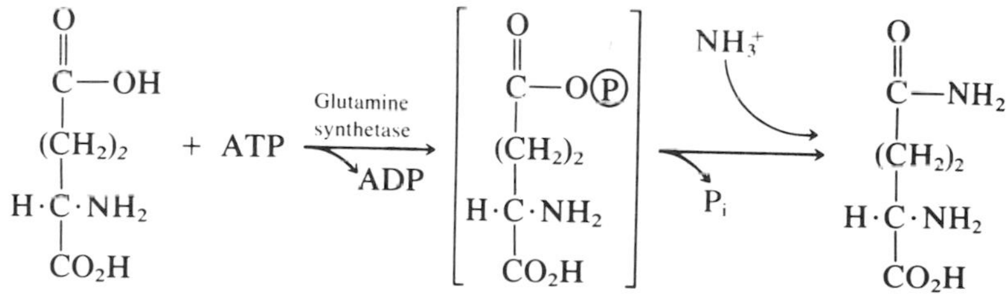

$$\begin{array}{c} O \\ \| \\ C-OH \\ | \\ (CH_2)_2 \\ | \\ H \cdot C \cdot NH_2 \\ | \\ CO_2H \end{array} + ATP \xrightarrow[\text{synthetase}]{\text{Glutamine}} ADP \left[\begin{array}{c} O \\ \| \\ C-O\text{\textcircled{P}} \\ | \\ (CH_2)_2 \\ | \\ H \cdot C \cdot NH_2 \\ | \\ CO_2H \end{array} \right] \xrightarrow[\text{P}_i]{NH_3^+} \begin{array}{c} O \\ \| \\ C-NH_2 \\ | \\ (CH_2)_2 \\ | \\ H \cdot C \cdot NH_2 \\ | \\ CO_2H \end{array}$$

Glutamate   Glutamine

$$\begin{array}{c} O \\ \| \\ C-NH_2 \\ | \\ (CH_2)_2 \\ | \\ H \cdot C \cdot NH_2 \\ | \\ CO_2H \end{array} + H_2O \xrightarrow{\text{Glutaminase}} \begin{array}{c} O \\ \| \\ C-OH \\ | \\ (CH_2)_2 \\ | \\ H \cdot C \cdot NH_2 \\ | \\ CO_2H \end{array} + NH_3$$

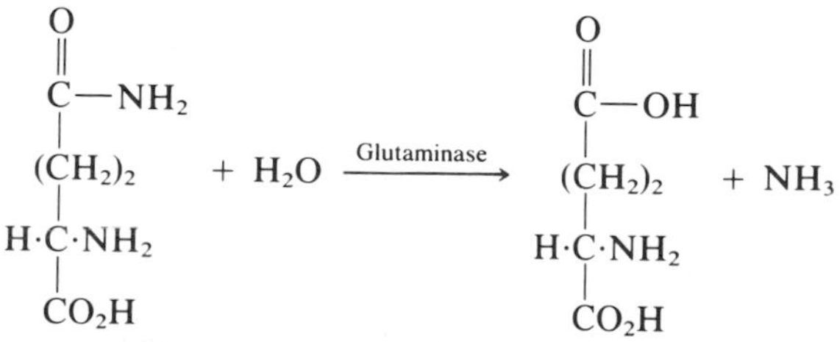

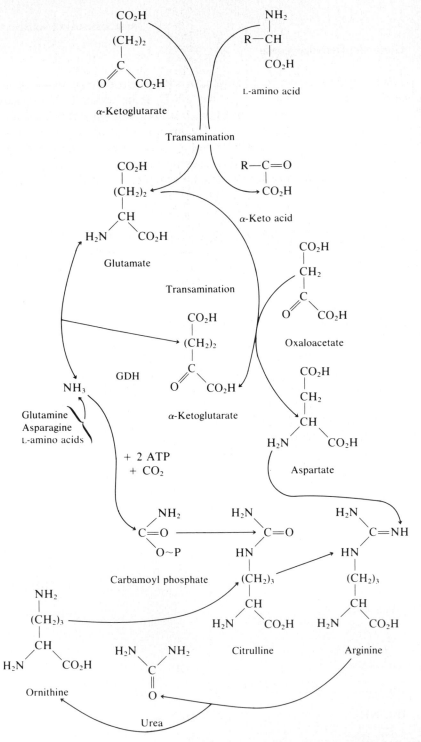

Fig. 5–2. *Transfer of amino groups from amino acids and ammonia to carbamoyl phosphate and the urea cycle.*

mine is of great importance metabolically as the donor of amino groups in a number of biosynthetic reactions such as the synthesis of purines and the conversion of uridine triphosphate (UTP) to cytidine triphosphate (CTP). In the synthesis of glutamine, the γ-carboxyl of glutamate is activated by reacting with the terminal phosphate of ATP to form γ-glutamyl phosphate. The phosphate is then replaced by ammonia and glutamine results.

Many cell membranes and the blood–brain barrier are relatively impermeable to glutamate; they are much more freely permeable to glutamine, which has no net charge at neutral pH. Tissues other than the liver probably receive the glutamate they need in the form of glutamine. The concentration of glutamine in the blood is relatively high, about 10^{-3}M, and it is even higher in tissues, about 10^{-2}M.

Urinary ammonia is derived from glutamine in the kidney, which has a high concentration of glutaminase. This enzyme hydrolyzes the glutamine that reaches the kidney from the blood. It cleaves glutamine to ammonia, which is excreted, and glutamate, which is reused. In a sense, glutamine is the storage and transport form of ammonia. Because ammonia is a very toxic substance, its concentration in the blood must be kept at a low level. During acidosis, the activity of kidney glutaminase and the excretion of ammonia in the urine increases. Normally, only about 2% to 5% of the total urinary nitrogen is ammonium ion, NH_4^+; in severe acidosis, however, as much as 50% may be ammonium ion. Even small increases in the concentration of ammonia in the blood lead to symptoms of a toxic response. This may be a factor in the onset of hepatic coma that results from the destruction of liver tissue associated with cirrhosis. The blood normally contains only 0.1 to 0.2 mg ammonia nitrogen per 100 ml, which is about 2×10^{-5}M. Ammonia interferes with neural transmission and may decrease the rate of the tricarboxylic acid cycle by funneling α-ketoglutarate to glutamate.

Because of the high toxicity of ammonia, several metabolic mechanisms have evolved to prevent its accumulation in tissues. One is the synthesis of urea. Neutral and nontoxic, urea is the principal nitrogen-containing waste product excreted by the human. It is the major end product of the metabolism of amino groups, and it is excreted at the rate of 10 to 25 g/day, depending on the amount of protein in the diet. The liver is the principal site of urea synthesis; therefore, liver disease or any condition that damages the liver decreases the person's ability to convert amino groups to urea. The concentration of amino acids in the blood remains elevated for a longer period of time.

Removal of the kidneys of an experimental animal prevents the excretion of urea, and the concentration of urea in the blood rises quickly. If the liver is removed and the kidneys are left intact, the concentration of urea in the blood falls. Urea is being excreted, but not produced. When both kidneys and liver are removed, the concentration of urea in the blood remains constant; it is being neither formed nor excreted.

Current understanding of urea synthesis began in 1932 when Sir Hans Krebs and a medical student, Kurt Henseleit, incubated liver slices in a medium containing ammonium salts, bicarbonate, and lactate as a source of energy. They added a variety of intermediate substances and measured the rate of urea production. The addition of ornithine, citrulline, or arginine to the liver slices greatly increased the production of urea. Ornithine and citrulline acted catalytically; that is, they increased the rate of urea synthesis, but were not used up in the process.

It had been known that the liver contains an arginase that converts arginine to urea and ornithine. Krebs and Henseleit postulated that urea is produced by a cyclic process involving the combination of ornithine, carbon dioxide, and ammonia to form citrulline, and the combination of citrulline with another mol of ammonia to form arginine. Finally, the hydrolytic splitting of arginine yields urea, making ornithine available to begin another turn of the cycle. This was the first cyclic process postulated in intermediary metabolism, and it antedated the tricarboxylic acid cycle by some years.

The overall cyclic process postulated by Krebs and Henseleit has been shown to be correct, but each step has been shown to be a complex process. The cyclic process is endergonic and requires some 28 kcal free energy per mol of urea synthesized. Neither carbon dioxide nor ammonia as such reacts with ornithine. Instead, the formation of citrulline involves the condensation of ornithine with carbamoyl phosphate, synthesized from carbon dioxide, ammonia, and ATP in a reaction that requires N-acetyl-glutamate as an allosteric activator.

Carbamoyl Phosphate

The formation of carbamoyl phosphate for urea synthesis occurs in the mitochondria. Some tissues have in the cytosol a different carbamoyl phosphate synthetase that catalyzes the production of carbamoyl phosphate to be used in the synthesis of pyrimidines. In the synthesis of carbamoyl phosphate in the mitochondria, bicarbonate is activated by ATP and converted to a carboxy phosphate bound to the enzyme:

$$\text{Enzyme} + \text{ATP} + \text{HCO}_3^- \rightarrow \text{Enzyme} - [^-\text{OCOOPO}_3^{2-}] + \text{ADP}$$

This reacts with NH_4^+ to form an enzyme-bound carbamate with the liberation of inorganic phosphate:

$$\text{Enzyme} - \left[^-\text{OCOOPO}_3^{2-}\right] + \text{NH}_4^+ \rightarrow \text{Enzyme} - \{\text{NH}_2 \cdot \text{COO}^-\} + \text{P}_i$$

A second ATP reacts to form carbamoyl phosphate, ADP, and the enzyme:

$$\text{Enzyme} - \left[\text{NH}_2 \cdot \text{COO}^-\right] + \text{ATP} \rightarrow \text{Enzyme} + \text{ADP} + \text{NH}_2\text{COOPO}_3^{2-}$$

$$\text{Sum:} \quad \text{NH}_4^+ + \text{HCO}_3^- + 2\,\text{ATP} \rightarrow \underset{\text{O}}{\overset{\text{NH}_2}{\underset{\textcircled{P}}{}}} \rangle\text{C}=\text{O} + 2\,\text{ADP} + \text{P}_i$$

The ammonia for the production of carbamoyl phosphate arises within the mitochondria by the oxidative deamination of glutamate catalyzed by glutamic dehydrogenase:

Glutamate $+$ NAD $+$ H_2O $\rightarrow$

α-Ketoglutarate $+$ NH_4^+ $+$ NADH $+$ H^+

Urea Cycle

The carbamoyl phosphate produced in the mitochondria donates the carbamoyl group to ornithine, which is formed in the cytosol but enters the mitochondrion by a special liver membrane transport system (Fig. 5–3). The condensation of ornithine and carbamoyl phosphate yields citrulline and inorganic phosphate, a reaction catalyzed by ornithine carbamoyl transferase. The citrulline leaves the mitochondrial compartment and passes into the cytosol of the liver cell.

The second amino group required for the synthesis of urea is derived not from ammonia, but from the amino group of aspartic acid. In a reaction driven by ATP and catalyzed by argininosuccinate synthetase in the cytosol, aspartic acid condenses with citrulline. The products are argininosuccinate, adenosine monophosphate (AMP), and inorganic pyrophosphate. The pyrophosphate formed in this reaction is hydrolyzed by pyrophosphatase to inorganic phosphate, thus pulling the overall reaction to the right.

The argininosuccinate is cleaved by argininosuccinate lyase, yielding free arginine and fumarate. The arginine is the immediate precursor of urea; it is hydrolyzed by arginase to form ornithine and urea. The fumarate is returned to the pool of intermediates in the tricarboxylic acid cycle, where it can be converted first to malate and then to oxaloacetate by the reactions of this cycle. Oxaloacetate can undergo transamination to yield aspartate, which is then available for the synthesis of another mole of argininosuccinate. Thus the Krebs–Henseleit urea cycle can be geared with the Krebs tricarboxylic acid cycle, forming what has been dubbed the Krebs "bicycle."

Only ammonia and carbon dioxide actually pass through the cycle. One of the amino groups of urea enters as carbamoyl phosphate; the other enters as the amino group of aspartate. The overall reaction can be written:

NH_4^+ $+$ CO_2 $+$ 3 ATP $+$ 2 H_2O $+$ Aspartate $\rightarrow$

Fumarate $+$ Urea $+$ 2 ADP $+$ 2 P_i $+$ AMP $+$ PP_i

The formation of one molecule of urea requires the hydrolysis of four energy-rich phosphate groups provided by ATP, approximately 28 kcal/mol urea synthesized.

Inherited Enzyme Deficiencies

Genetic defects of enzymes involved in the urea cycle lead to mental retardation. Patients with such defects may be treated by giving in the diet the α-keto acids that correspond to the essential amino acids. The essential parts of the essential amino acids are the carbon chains, which cannot be synthesized by human tissues.

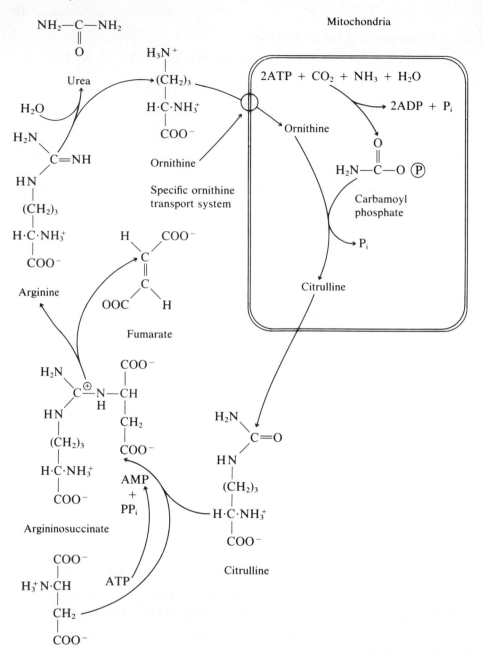

Fig. 5–3. *The urea cycle. Carbamoyl phosphate, made from CO_2 and NH_3 in the mitochondria, unites with ornithine to form citrulline, which then leaves the mitochondria, gains an amino group from aspartate, and forms arginine. Arginase splits arginine and releases urea, leaving ornithine free to return to the mitochondria and begin a new cycle.*

These α-keto analogs can accept amino groups from other amino acids by transamination and, in this way, decrease the overall production of free ammonia.

HYPERAMMONEMIA

Elevated levels of ammonia in tissues, blood, and urine result from the lack of either carbamoyl phosphate synthetase or ornithine carbamoyl transferase. Infants with hyperammonemia have episodic vomiting and irritability that progresses to lethargy, coma, and convulsions. There is some clinical improvement if the patient is fed a diet low in protein (1.5 g/kg body weight per day). In a normal individual, the ammonia content in the plasma is about 55 μg/100 ml; in patients with hyperammonemia, the concentration may be as high as 1,000 or 1,200 μg/100 ml. The excretion of pyrimidine metabolites may also be increased in these patients.

CITRULLINEMIA

Elevated levels of citrulline in tissues, blood, and urine result from a deficiency of argininosuccinate synthetase. Urea is excreted in nearly normal amounts, perhaps because the brain lacks a specific isoenzyme of argininosuccinate synthetase whereas the liver contains its specific isoenzyme and produces urea at the normal rate.

ARGININOSUCCINIC ACIDEMIA

A deficiency of argininosuccinate lyase results in elevated levels of argininosuccinate in tissues and blood. As in citrullinemia, urea is excreted in nearly normal amounts, and it is postulated that the condition may be caused by the lack of a specific isoenzyme in the brain and the normal presence of a different isoenzyme in the liver.

METABOLISM OF METHIONINE AND CYSTEINE

The amount of sulfur taken in and excreted by an adult human is relatively constant, about 0.7 g/day on the usual diet. Sulfur appears in the urine as inorganic sulfate (about 80% of the total), organic sulfur (about 15%), and ester sulfate (about 5%). Ester sulfate is sulfur esterified with an alcohol, such as phenol or indoxyl.

Methionine is an essential amino acid. Of key importance is its reaction with ATP to form S-adenosyl methionine, which is a donor of methyl groups and other compounds in biochemical reactions (Fig. 5–4). The compound remaining after transfer of the methyl group is S-adenosyl homocysteine. This is hydrolyzed to homocysteine, which reacts with serine to form cystathionine. Patients with severe liver necrosis may have a reduced ability to use methionine. It then accumulates and serves as a substrate for thionase, which normally cleaves cystathionine. Thio-

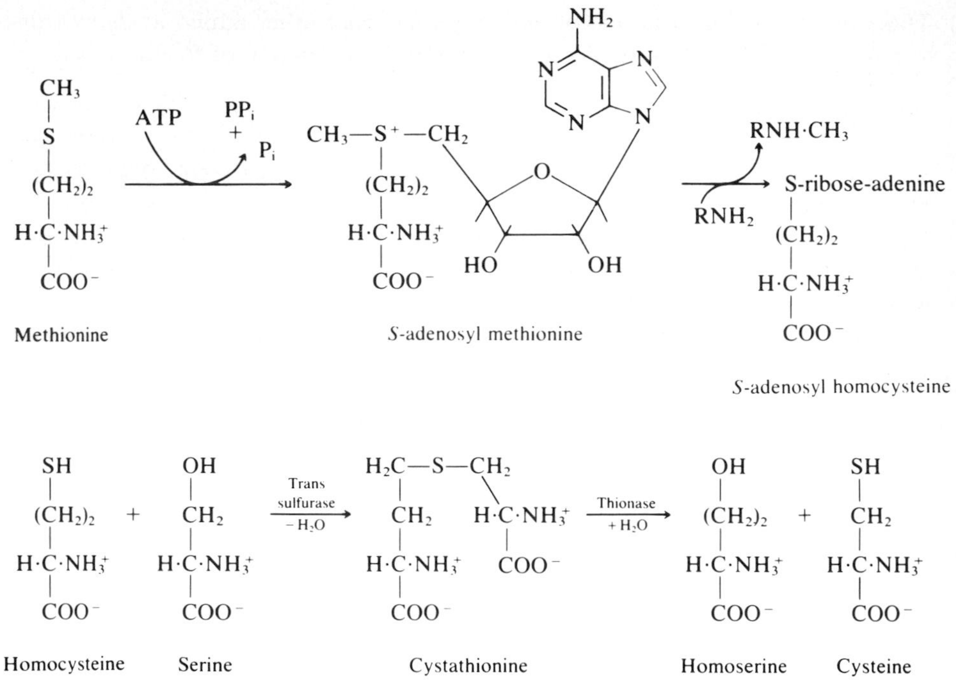

Fig. 5–4. *Metabolism of methionine. The methyl group of* S-*adenosyl methionine can be transferred to any of several acceptors (RNH·CH₃). The sulfur of homocysteine may be transferred via cystathionine to form cysteine.*

nase cleaves methionine to homoserine and methyl mercaptan, CH_3SH, which contributes to the foul odor, called fetor hepaticus, of the breath and urine of patients with liver necrosis.

Cystathionine is present in high concentrations in nervous tissues, especially in the brain of primates, where its concentration approaches 50 mg/100g tissue. Normally, cystathionine is cleaved by thionase to yield homoserine and cysteine. These reactions transfer the sulfur originally present in methionine to the sulfur of cysteine. Neither cysteine nor its dimer, cystine, are essential amino acids, since they can be produced in the body from methionine and serine. In the biosynthesis of cysteine, the carbon chain and the amino group are derived from serine, but the sulfur is derived from methionine. When ^{15}N-labeled serine is fed to rats, a large fraction of the ^{15}N can be isolated from the cystine in the tissues. When methionine labeled with ^{35}S and with ^{14}C in its carbon chain is fed to a rabbit, the cystine in the hair proteins contains a great deal of ^{35}S, but very little, if any, ^{14}C. Cystine and cysteine are interconvertible by a reaction involving glutathione. The carbon chain of cysteine is converted to pyruvate, and the sulfur is removed and excreted as inorganic sulfate.

As an alternative, the sulfate may react with ATP to form phosphoadenosine phosphosulfate (PAPS), the donor of sulfate groups in the synthesis of complex mucopolysaccharides and in the conjugation of steroids. Cysteine sulfinate, an intermediate in the breakdown of cysteine, may be converted to taurine by oxidative decarboxylative reactions. The taurine may react with cholyl CoA to form taurocholic acid, one of the bile acids important in promoting the digestion and absorption of fats.

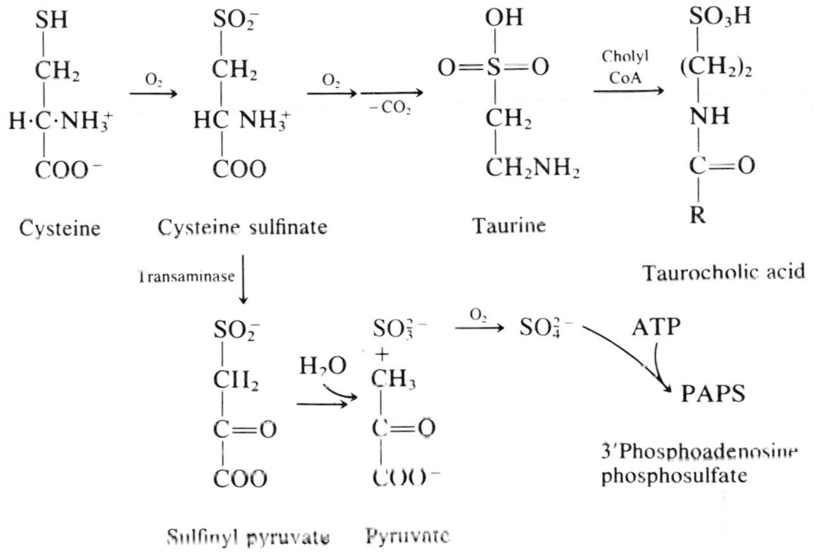

$$
\begin{array}{ccccccc}
\text{SH} & & \text{SO}_2^- & & \text{OH} & & \text{SO}_3\text{H} \\
| & & | & & | & & | \\
\text{CH}_2 & \xrightarrow{\text{O}_2} & \text{CH}_2 & \xrightarrow[-\text{CO}_2]{\text{O}_2} & \text{O}=\text{S}=\text{O} & \xrightarrow{\substack{\text{Cholyl}\\\text{CoA}}} & (\text{CH}_2)_2 \\
| & & | & & | & & | \\
\text{H}\cdot\text{C}\cdot\text{NH}_3^+ & & \text{HC NH}_3^+ & & \text{CH}_2 & & \text{NH} \\
| & & | & & | & & | \\
\text{COO}^- & & \text{COO} & & \text{CH}_2\text{NH}_2 & & \text{C}=\text{O} \\
& & & & & & | \\
\text{Cysteine} & & \text{Cysteine sulfinate} & & \text{Taurine} & & \text{R}
\end{array}
$$

Taurocholic acid

Transaminase ↓

$$
\begin{array}{ccccc}
\text{SO}_2^- & & \text{SO}_3^{2-} & \xrightarrow{\text{O}_2} \text{SO}_4^{2-} & \text{ATP} \\
| & \text{H}_2\text{O} & + & & \\
\text{CH}_2 & \longrightarrow & \text{CH}_3 & & \\
| & & | & & \searrow \\
\text{C}=\text{O} & & \text{C}=\text{O} & & \text{PAPS} \\
| & & | & & \\
\text{COO} & & \text{COO}^- & &
\end{array}
$$

3′Phosphoadenosine phosphosulfate

Sulfinyl pyruvate   Pyruvate

The ester sulfate fraction includes compounds in which inorganic sulfate is esterified with an alcohol (e.g., phenol or indoxyl). In synthesizing ester sulfate, the sulfate first reacts with ATP to form adenosine 5′-phosphosulfate. This reacts with a second mol of ATP to form 3-phosphoadenosine, 5′-phosphosulfate, (PAPS) which is the active form that donates a sulfur group.

Cystinuria

An inborn error of metabolism produces cystinuria, in which a significant quantity of cystine is excreted in the urine. This amino acid was discovered in 1810 when Wollaston, a member of the Royal Society of London, collected kidney stones and discovered that some of these contained uric acid, while others contained cystine. Cystinurics may excrete as much as 2 g cystine per day.

Cystinurics excrete more organic sulfate and much less inorganic sulfate than normal persons do. Nearly half the sulfur they excrete is in the form of cystine. It had been thought that cystinuria must be caused by the lack of some enzyme involved in the oxidation of cysteine to inorganic sulfate, but it was discovered that cystinurics also excrete a much greater than normal amount of α-amino nitrogen. In other words, they also excrete increased amounts of amino acids other than cystine. Cystinurics fed cystine labeled with ^{34}S, excrete not only labeled cystine, but also labeled inorganic sulfate, indicating that this is not simply a block in the oxidation of the cystine. Cystinurics excrete in the urine the amino acids lysine, arginine, and ornithine, as well as the diamines, putrescine (obtained by the decarboxylation of ornithine) and cadavarine (obtained by the decarboxylation of lysine). All these compounds have two amino groups, and it is now established that cystinurics suffer from the congenital absence of a specific transport system in the kidney tubule, a system that normally carries out the tubular reabsorption of these diamino compounds.

Because cystine is a relatively insoluble amino acid, cystinurics may develop kidney stones composed of cystine. They should be given a low protein diet, one with the smallest possible amounts of sulfur-containing amino acids, and should be given a great deal of water so that the cystine can be excreted in solution. It may be necessary to wake these patients in the middle of the night to give them more water so that cystine stones do not form during the night.

Cystinosis

Another inherited disease that involves the excretion of many different amino acids is cystinosis. It is characterized by the deposition of cystine as crystals in tissues throughout the body. An individual with cystinosis has retarded growth, a kind of rickets, a decreased level of serum phosphorus, osteomalacia, glycosuria, and a generalized amino aciduria. Cystinosis is a very serious disease; the decreased ability to use cystine appears to be one aspect of a more generalized disease called Fanconi's syndrome, which is characterized by defective renal tubular reabsorption of glucose, phosphate, and a variety of amino acids.

BRANCHED CHAIN AMINO ACIDS

Metabolism of Valine, Leucine, and Isoleucine

The three amino acids with branched aliphatic chains are valine, leucine, and isoleucine. Valine is glucogenic; leucine is the most ketogenic of all amino acids, since 1 mol leucine gives rise to 1.5 mol acetoacetate; and isoleucine is in part glucogenic and in part ketogenic. The initial steps in the metabolism of each of the three amino acids are very similar. Each first undergoes transamination with α-ketoglutarate to form the corresponding α-keto acid and then undergoes oxidative decarboxylation by reactions involving NAD, CoA, thiamine pyrophosphate, lipoic acid, and FAD. In other words, the reaction is very much like the oxidative decarboxylation of pyruvic acid and α-ketoglutaric acid. The product is the CoA derivative of an α-ketocarboxylic acid, one carbon shorter than the reactant (Fig. 5–5).

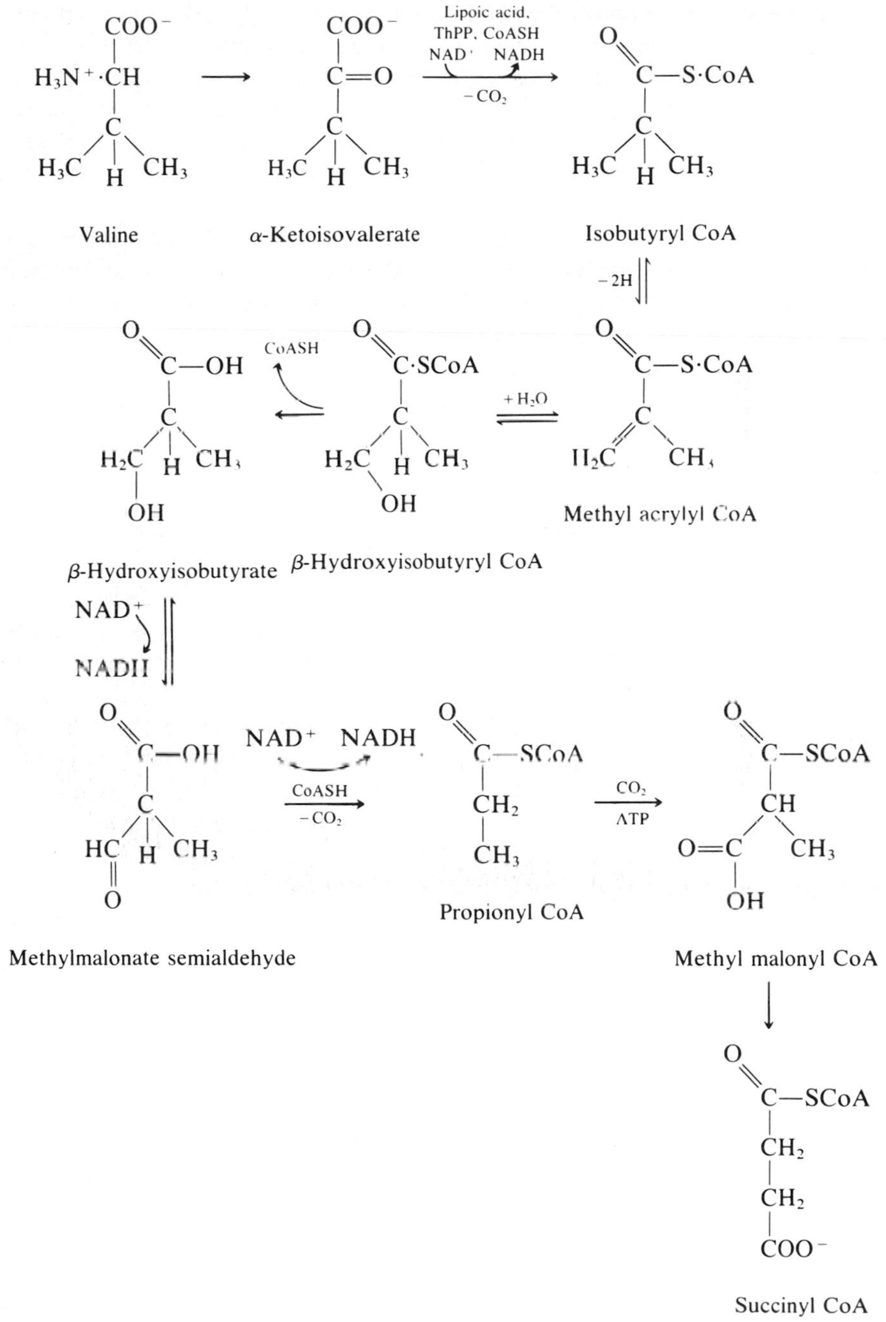

COO⁻ ⟶ COO⁻ $\xrightarrow[-CO_2]{\text{Lipoic acid, ThPP, CoASH} \atop \text{NAD}^+ \quad \text{NADH}}$ O
H₃N⁺·CH   C=O   C—S·CoA
   C   C   C
H₃C H CH₃   H₃C H CH₃   H₃C H CH₃

Valine   α-Ketoisovalerate   Isobutyryl CoA

-2H

O   O   O
C—OH ⟵CoASH⟵ C·SCoA ⇌+H₂O⇌   C—S·CoA
C   C   C
H₂C H CH₃   H₂C H CH₃   H₂C   CH₃
OH   OH   Methyl acrylyl CoA

β-Hydroxyisobutyrate β-Hydroxyisobutyryl CoA

NAD⁺
NADH

O   NAD⁺ NADH   O   O
C—OH $\xrightarrow[-CO_2]{\text{CoASH}}$ C—SCoA $\xrightarrow[\text{ATP}]{CO_2}$ C—SCoA
C   CH₂   CH
HC H CH₃   CH₃   O=C   CH₃
O   OH

Methylmalonate semialdehyde   Propionyl CoA   Methyl malonyl CoA

O
C—SCoA
CH₂
CH₂
COO⁻

Succinyl CoA

Fig. 5–5. *Metabolism of the branched-chain amino acid valine, indicating the reactions by which it yields succinyl CoA and hence is glucogenic.*

The metabolism of both valine and isoleucine eventually yields methyl malonyl CoA (Fig. 5–6). The methyl malonyl CoA undergoes a curious reaction that is catalyzed by a mutase and requires the vitamin B_{12} derivative cobalamin as a cofactor. The entire thioester group is transferred from one carbon to the next, yielding succinyl CoA. The succinyl CoA is then converted by way of the other dicarboxylic acids to phosphoenol pyruvate and ultimately yields glucose. Three of the five carbons of valine are glucogenic.

In the metabolism of isoleucine, one molecule of acetyl CoA (which is ketogenic) and one molecule of propionic acid as propionyl CoA is formed. Propionyl CoA is carboxylated to methyl malonyl CoA, and this is then metabolized by the mutase to succinyl CoA. Isoleucine is thus in part glucogenic and in part ketogenic. Leucine is converted by way of isovaleryl CoA and hydroxymethyl glutaryl CoA to acetoacetic acid plus an acetyl group. Thus all six carbons of leucine are converted to ketone bodies (Fig. 5–6).

Maple Syrup Urine Disease

A number of children have a genetic defect that causes the urine to have a characteristic and distinctive odor. The urinary constituents have been identified as the α-ketoacids corresponding to the aliphatic branched chain amino acids. Because it is alleged that the urine smells like maple syrup, the condition has been called "maple syrup urine" disease. The disease is disastrous, and infants who suffer from it have severe neurologic damage that becomes evident shortly after birth; the infants typically die within a few weeks. By restricting the dietary intake of these three amino acids, however, it has been possible to prolong the life of these infants considerably.

Studies of these infants show that they have the transaminases in normal amounts, but the oxidative decarboxylation to the acyl CoA does not occur. Initially, it was inferred from these findings that all three α-keto acids are dehydrogenated by a common enzyme and that there is no major alternative pathway. It now appears that one enzyme, ketoisocaproate dehydrogenase, catalyzes the oxidative decarboxylation of the keto acids corresponding to leucine and isoleucine, but a different enzyme, ketoisovalerate dehydrogenase, catalyzes the oxidative decarboxylation of ketoisovalerate derived from valine. Because the high concentrations of keto acid analogs of leucine and isoleucine inhibit this enzyme, ketoisovalerate accumulates. These three keto acids with their corresponding amino acids damage the brain and interfere markedly with the function of the nervous system.

Isovaleric Acidemia and Jamaican Vomiting Disease

A rare defect of the metabolism of leucine causes isovaleric acidemia, which results when isovaleryl CoA is not oxidized. This condition is often fatal. Patients

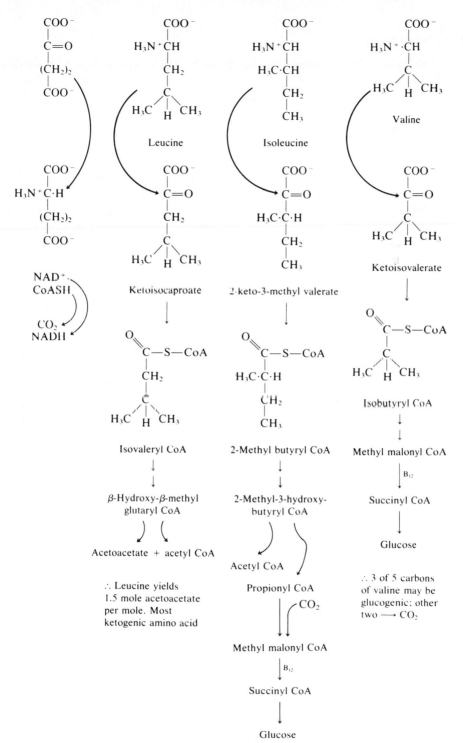

Fig. 5–6. *Metabolism of branched-chain amino acids comparing glucogenic and ketogenic amino acids.*

have a characteristic odor, described as "cheesy" or "like sweaty feet." This is due to the branched chain compounds. Patients can be treated by feeding them excess glycine, since glycine reacts with isovaleryl CoA to form isovaleryl glycine, which is excreted in the urine.

Comparable symptoms are associated with Jamaican vomiting disease, caused by eating the unripe fruit of the ackee tree. This fruit contains an unusual amino acid called hypoglycin A, L-2 amino, 3-methylene cyclopropyl propionic acid. This undergoes oxidative deamination to yield methylene cyclopropyl acetic acid, which specifically inhibits isovaleryl CoA dehydrogenase, thereby causing an accumulation of isovaleric acid in the blood that can reach a concentration 50-fold over normal. Isovalerate is very toxic and accounts for some of the symptoms of the disease, such as vomiting, convulsions, and coma. The accompanying depression of the CNS may be due to the accumulation of the isovaleric acid in the blood. The cause of death is probably hypoglycemia, however, for the blood glucose levels may fall to as low as 10% of the normal concentration.

By interfering with the transport of long-chain fatty acids into the mitochondria, a process that requires carnitine, hypoglycin interferes with the oxidation of these fatty acids. Thus a major source of the body's supply of energy is eliminated. The metabolism of glucose is greatly increased to make up for this deficit of energy. After the readily available supply of blood glucose and liver glycogen has been exhausted, the patient becomes hypoglycemic and may die. In Jamaica, ackee fruit is typically cooked up with salt codfish. The proteins in salt codfish contain a great deal of leucine, and the leucine contributes to the accumulation of isovaleric acid that cannot be metabolized further because of the inhibition of isovaleryl CoA dehydrogenase. Thus the blocking of isovaleryl CoA dehydrogenase can result from either an inborn error, such as that in isovaleric acidemia, or an environmental toxin, such as that in Jamaican vomiting disease.

HETEROCYCLIC AMINO ACIDS

Metabolism of Tryptophan

An essential amino acid, tryptophan is metabolized in one of two pathways. One involves in its first step a transformation to 5-hydroxytryptophan (Fig. 5–7). This is catalyzed by tryptophan monooxygenase, an enzyme that requires tetrahydropteridine as its reductant cofactor. This is related to tetrahydrofolic acid, but is a pteridine ring without the para-aminobenzoic acid and glutamate. A similar cofactor is involved in the hydroxylation of phenylalanine to tyrosine which we will discuss a little later. 5-Hydroxytryptophan undergoes decarboxylation to 5-hydroxytryptamine, also known as serotonin, a potent vasoconstrictor found especially in the brain, in Mast cells, and in blood platelets. A constituent of wasp venom and toad venom, it is a neurohumoral agent in human beings. Some drugs that have marked effects on the CNS, such as LSD, are potent antagonists of serotonin. 5-Hydroxytryptamine is oxidized to 5-hydroxyindoleacetic acid and excreted as such. About 3% of the tryptophan in the diet is metabolized to serotonin and excreted as 5-hydroxyindoleacetic acid.

The major pathway of tryptophan degradation is its oxidation to kynurenine by way of an intermediate N-formyl kynurenine, a reaction catalyzed by tryptophan-2,3-dioxygenase (Fig. 5–7). The control of tryptophan dioxygenase has been investigated extensively. The enzyme is not present in the livers of fetal and newborn rats until the tenth postnatal day, although its appearance can be induced prematurely by the administration of adrenocortical steroids. After day 10, the administration of either a glucocorticoid or the substrate, tryptophan, increases the level of enzymatic activity. The elevation of enzyme activity that follows steroid administration occurs because the synthesis of the specific messenger RNA that codes for the synthesis of the dioxygenase is stimulated. In contrast, the increased levels of dioxygenase activity induced by the administration of additional dietary tryptophan result from a decreased rate of degradation of the enzyme; the synthesis of the enzyme proceeds at the normal rate.

The oxygen that is added enters as molecular oxygen, which attacks and opens the pyrrol ring, forming N-formyl kynurenine. The formyl group is removed by a formamidase, and the resulting kynurenine undergoes an additional hydroxylation that uses NADPH and molecular oxygen, and results in the formation of 3-hydroxykynurenine. This undergoes a cleavage catalyzed by the enzyme kynureninase to yield 3-hydroxyanthranilic acid and alanine. By a series of reactions, 3-hydroxyanthranilic acid can be converted into nicotinic acid (which is usually considered a vitamin), and nicotinic acid can be converted to NAD. The lessened growth rate of niacin-deficient rats can be returned to normal by administering tryptophan.

In Hartnup's disease, a hereditary disorder associated with mental retardation, only a small fraction of ingested tryptophan is oxidized. This is not because of any defect in the enzymes that metabolize tryptophan, however, but rather because of a defect in the intestinal and renal transport of amino acids. Hartnup's disease is due to a defect in the mechanism for the reabsorption of neutral amino acids that results in the excessive excretion of these amino acids in the urine, thus decreasing the concentration of the amino acid in blood and tissues and, hence, decreasing production of nicotinamide or niacin by these pathways. Patients with Hartnup's disease exhibit specific symptoms, skin rashes, neurologic and mental disturbances that are similar to those of patients with pellagra. The discovery that Hartnup patients respond to oral nicotinamide therapy led to the conclusion that the symptoms were due to a relative deficiency of tryptophan. The symptoms do not appear unless the dietary supply of nicotinamide is low. During rapid growth, when there is a greater requirement for nicotinamide, the symptoms tend to be exacerbated. Later, when the growth period is completed, the patients tend to improve clinically.

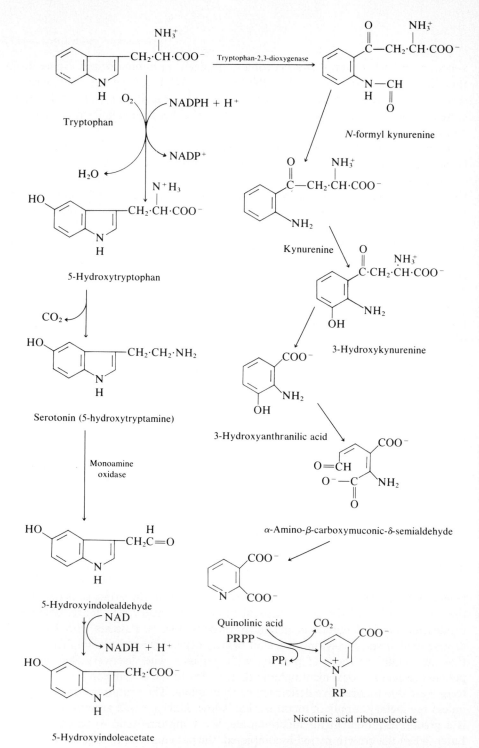

Fig. 5–7. *Aspects of the metabolism of tryptophan: Its conversion to serotonin, kynurenine, and nicotinic acid.*

Metabolism of Histidine

An essential amino acid for the growth of young animals, histidine is unique among amino acids in that it contains the imidazole ring. When ^{15}N-labeled ammonia is fed to rats, the histidine of the tissue proteins contains ^{15}N in the α-amino group (transferred by transamination), but the nitrogens in the imidazole ring are not labeled. This is one indication that the animal body cannot synthesize the imidazole ring. Histidine is converted in the liver to urocanic acid, a reaction catalyzed by the enzyme histidase (Fig. 5–8). The enzyme urocanase splits the

Fig. 5–8. *Metabolism of histidine to histamine and glutamate.*

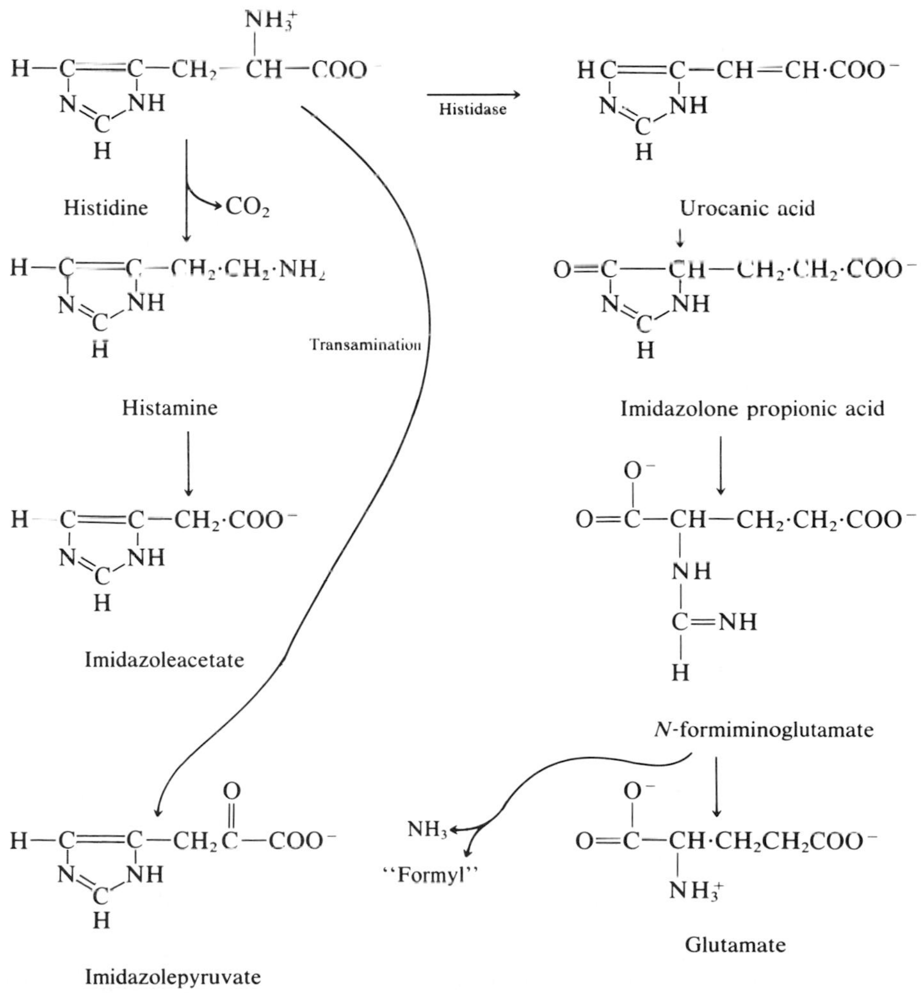

imidazole ring, producing formiminoglutamic acid. The formimino group is transferred to tetrahydrofolic acid, and the remainder of the molecule is glutamic acid. Thus, histidine is a glucogenic amino acid.

In an alternative pathway, histidine undergoes decarboxylation to yield histamine, a reaction catalyzed by histidine decarboxylase. Histamine is formed in the lung, liver, muscle, gastric mucosa, and other tissues. The histidine decarboxylase in Mast cells converts histidine to histamine and accounts for the high content of histamine in these cells. Histamine is a powerful vasodilator and vasodepressant. Finally, the enzyme histaminase or diamine oxidase converts histamine to β-imidazole acetic acid.

Histidine is a constituent of two dipeptides found in muscle. Carnosine is β-alanyl histidine, and anserine is β-alanyl, 1-methyl histidine.

Histidinemia, the elevated level of histidine in the blood, is accompanied by an increased excretion of histidine in the urine. Patients with this disorder commonly have mental retardation and speech impairment, although some histidinemic patients have normal intelligence. In addition to increased concentrations of histidine, the concentration of imidazole–pyruvic acid is increased in the urine. This compound is an aryl substituted pyruvic acid and resembles phenylpyruvic acid enough to give the urine of affected individuals the characteristic green color with ferric chloride that is a test of phenylketonuria. The elevated level of urinary imidazole–pyruvic acid suggests that the defect is in the histidine ammonia lyase or histidase. This can be confirmed by enzymatic assay of biopsy samples. The product of histidase, urocanic acid, is present in the sweat of normal individuals, but it is absent from the sweat of histidinemic patients. Imidazole–pyruvic acid is formed by the transamination of histidine; normally, this is a minor pathway of histidine degradation.

METABOLISM OF PHENYLALANINE AND TYROSINE

Phenylalanine is an essential amino acid in mammals; because it can be formed from phenylalanine, tyrosine is not essential. Phenylalanine can be converted to tyrosine, but the reverse reaction does not occur. The hydroxylation of phenylalanine to tyrosine is catalyzed by phenylalanine hydroxylase, a mixed function oxidase so-called because one atom of oxygen appears in the product and the other appears in water. The reaction requires molecular oxygen; NADPH; and a cofactor, an electron carrier called tetrahydrobiopterin or tetrahydropteridine. Phenylalanine reacts with oxygen and with 5,6,7,8-tetrahydropteridine to form tyrosine. In a second reaction, 7,8-dihydropteridine reacts with NADPH to yield 5,6,7,8-tetrahydropteridine and oxidized $NADP^+$, a reaction catalyzed by dihydropteridine reductase. The sum of these reactions is

$$\text{Phenylalanine} + O_2 + \text{NADPH} + H^+ \rightarrow \text{Tyrosine} + NADP^+ + H_2O$$

Tyrosine is the precursor of a number of compounds of biologic and medical importance: the catecholamines, epinephrine and norepinephrine; melanin, the black pigment in the skin; and thyroxine, the hormone produced by the thyroid gland (Fig. 5–9). Tyrosine is metabolized by a pathway that leads to the production of fumarate and acetoacetate so that tyrosine and phenylalanine are in part glucogenic and in part ketogenic.

Production of Catecholamines

Tyrosine is hydroxylated to 3,4-dihydroxyphenylalanine, and this, in turn, is decarboxylated to yield 3,4-dihydroxyphenyl ethylamine. This is hydroxylated to norepinephrine, and norepinephrine accepts a methyl group from S-adenosyl methionine to become epinephrine. These two vasoactive compounds, epinephrine and norepinephrine, are catecholamines. Each contains a benzene ring with two hydroxyl groups (catechol), and each has an amine group at the opposite end of the molecule.

Melanin and Albinism

In the basal layer of the epidermis are cells called melanoblasts in which the dark pigment, melanin, is synthesized from tyrosine by a copper-containing enzyme called tyrosinase. This enzyme catalyzes the oxidation of tyrosine to dihydroxyphenylalanine (dopa) and to dopa quinone. The ring of the dopa quinone undergoes closure to yield indol-5,6-quinone, and this is polymerized to form melanins. Complex substances of high molecular weight, melanins are insoluble in most solvents. In tissues, they are usually combined with protein. In these oxidations, the product of one reaction, 3,4-dihydroxyphenylalanine, is the hydrogen donor for the second reaction, which produces phenylalanine-3,4-quinone. The tanning of human skin is initiated by the ultraviolet irradiation of tyrosine, which leads to the formation of dihydroxyphenylalanine.

The total lack of melanin is termed albinism. An albino may not have the melanin-forming cells or the tyrosinase necessary to convert phenylalanine to phenylalanine-3,4-quinone. In the absence of this enzyme, no melanin is formed in the skin, the hair, or the iris of the eye, and the individual has dead white skin and pink eyes. Albinos can synthesize epinephrine and norepinephrine, however, which indicates that a different kind of tyrosinase is involved in the synthesis of dihydroxyphenylalanine in the adrenal medulla and CNS.

Biosynthesis of Thyroxine

The active hormone of the thyroid gland, thyroxine, is synthesized from tyrosine while the tyrosine is bound in a large protein molecule called thyroglobulin. Tyrosine has iodine added to it to form first monoiodotyrosine, then diiodotyrosine. Two molecules of diiodotyrosine are coupled together to form thyroxine.

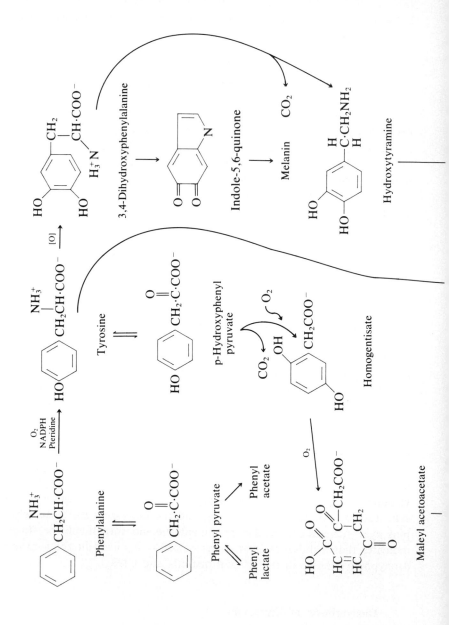

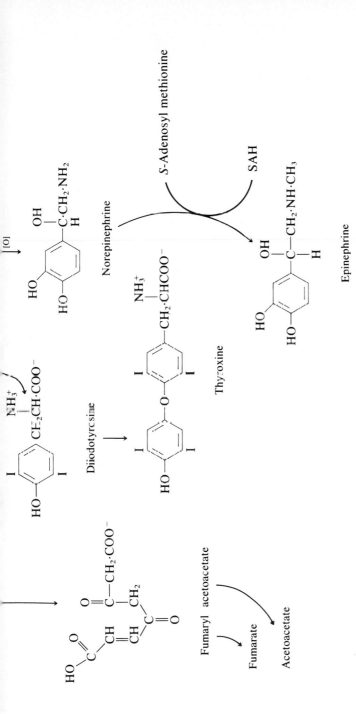

Fig. 5–9. *Metabolism of phenylalanine and tyrosine, illustrating the production of melanin, thyroxine, and epinephrine.*

Phenylketonuria and Mental Retardation

The initial event in the metabolism of tyrosine is a transamination catalyzed by tyrosine glutamate amino transferase. This enzyme is inducible; its synthesis is increased significantly in the liver after the administration of its substrate tyrosine or of adrenocortical steroids.

The activity of this enzyme is decreased following the injection of somatotropin (growth hormone) secreted by the pituitary. A copper-containing protein, p-hydroxyphenyl pyruvate dioxygenase catalyzes the oxidation of p-hydroxyphenyl pyruvate to homogentisic acid. This is a very complex reaction that involves hydroxylation of the ring, oxidation, decarboxylation, and migration of the side chain. Ascorbic acid is in some way essential for the normal activity of this hydroxyphenyl pyruvate dioxygenase. The next step, the oxidation of homogentisic acid, is catalyzed by homogentisic dioxygenase, which requires ferrous iron and reduced glutathione for its action. The aromatic ring is cut between the side chain and the adjacent hydroxyl group; one of the oxygen atoms becomes the 3-carbonyl oxygen of the product, maleyl acetoacetate, and the other becomes the carbonyl oxygen of the carboxyl group.

In phenylketonuria (PKU), phenylalanine hydroxylase is deficient. A phenylketonuric excretes as much as 1 or 2 g phenylpyruvic acid per day in the urine, as well as increased quantities of phenylalanine and phenyl lactic acid. The ability of the liver to convert phenylalanine to tyrosine is reduced to 10% or less of the normal rate. Phenylketonurics usually have decreased pigmentation in the skin, since phenylalanine is not being converted to tyrosine at the usual rate and is less available as a precursor of melanin. The concentration of phenylalanine in the blood and tissues increases, and the mental deficiency associated with PKU is due to the accumulation of phenylalanine and its metabolites in the CNS.

The condition is inherited as a recessive mendelian trait. About 1 person in 60 is heterozygous for this gene, and 1 person in 15,000 is homozygous and shows PKU. About 1% of all the people institutionalized with mental retardation suffer from PKU. If this condition is diagnosed immediately in a newborn and the neonate is placed on a dietary regime low in phenylalanine, the severity of the resulting mental deficiency can be greatly decreased.

There are several other types of hyperphenylalaninemia. One is due to a defect in the dihydropteridine reductase, the enzyme that catalyzes the regeneration of tetrahydropteridine to serve as cofactor for phenylalanine hydroxylase. Unlike patients with PKU, these patients demonstrate symptoms shortly after birth and do not respond to the standard dietary treatment of reduced phenylalanine intake.

Alkaptonuria

In alkaptonuria, a rare metabolic condition, the patient lacks homogentisic dioxygenase. The urine of an alkaptonuric turns dark on contact with air, since homogentisic acid undergoes polymerization, resulting in a melaninlike material that is insoluble in water. Homogentisic acid is a strongly reducing material that gives a violet color with dilute ferric chloride. Like PKU, alkaptonuria is inherited as a recessive mendelian trait. In early life, no abnormality other than the darkening of the urine is apparent, but in later years, there may be abnormal deposition of pigments in cartilage, tendons, and fibrous tissues.

GLYCINE AND ITS METABOLISM

Like other amino acids, glycine may be activated and joined to its specific transfer RNA to be incorporated into peptide chains. In addition, glycine serves as the precursor of a portion of the purine ring and is incorporated into creatine phosphate (an energy-rich phosphate compound in muscle), as well as into the porphyrin ring in hemoglobin and the cytochromes.

Glycine plays other metabolic roles in detoxification reactions. Benzoic acid, a slightly soluble compound added to many foods as a preservative, is prevented from accumulating by conversion to benzoyl CoA and reaction with glycine to form benzoyl glycine, also called hippuric acid, which is much more soluble and more easily excreted. Glycine is also a precursor and component of the tripeptide glutathione, γ-glutamyl cysteinyl glycine, which plays important roles in oxidation–reduction reactions.

Creatine Phosphate

A succession of transfer reactions synthesizes creatine phosphate. In the first, an amidine group is transferred from arginine to glycine, forming guanidinoacetate and leaving ornithine. In a sense, glycine cleaves arginine much as water cleaves arginine in the arginase reaction. Ornithine may enter the urea cycle and lead to the production of another molecule of arginine.

$$
\begin{array}{c}
\underset{\text{Glycine}}{
\begin{array}{c}
NH_3^+ \\
| \\
CH_2 \\
| \\
COO^-
\end{array}}
\;+\;
\underset{\text{Arginine}}{
\begin{array}{c}
H_2N \;\overset{+}{\underset{}{\diagup}}\; NH_2 \\
C \\
| \\
NH \\
| \\
(CH_2)_3 \\
| \\
H \cdot C \cdot NH_3^+ \\
| \\
COO^-
\end{array}}
\;\longrightarrow\;
\underset{\text{Guanidinoacetate}}{
\begin{array}{c}
H_2N \;\overset{+}{\underset{}{\diagup}}\; NH_2 \\
C \\
| \\
NH \\
| \\
CH_2 \\
| \\
COO^-
\end{array}}
\;+\;
\underset{\text{Ornithine}}{
\begin{array}{c}
NH_3^+ \\
| \\
(CH_2)_3 \\
| \\
H \cdot C \cdot NH_3^+ \\
| \\
COO^-
\end{array}}
\end{array}
$$

Guanidinoacetate accepts a methyl group from *S*-adenosyl methionine, forming creatine and leaving *S*-adenosyl homocysteine. This transfer of the methyl group is an irreversible reaction.

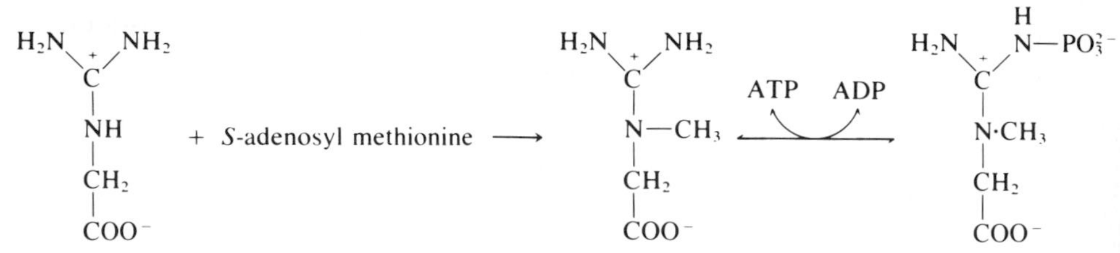

Guanidino acetate   Creatine   Phosphocreatine

Creatine is converted to creatine phosphate by the transfer of the terminal phosphate group from ATP. This reaction, catalyzed by creatine kinase, is readily reversible. The concentration of ATP in skeletal muscle is approximately 10^{-5} mol/kg. This is enough ATP for perhaps 0.2 second of strenuous muscular exercise. The amount of creatine phosphate in muscle is about 3×10^{-2} mol/kg, and this provides the energy for perhaps 30 seconds of strenuous muscular exercise. Thus, creatine phosphate serves as a depot for energy-rich phosphate groups within the muscle.

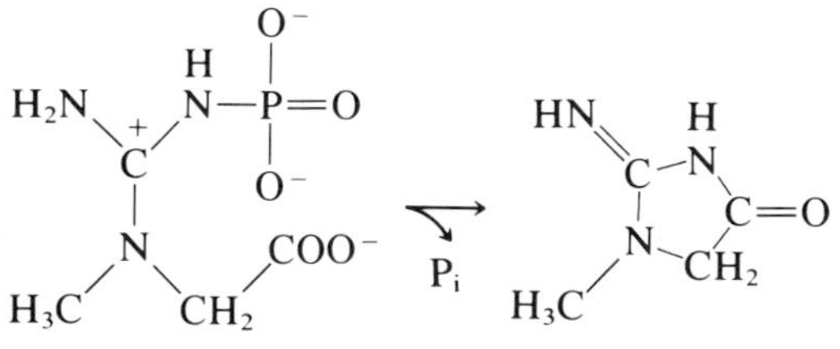

Creatine phosphate   Creatinine

Both creatine and creatine phosphate undergo a slow, spontaneous cyclization to form creatinine, which is excreted in the urine. The creatinine excreted amounts to about 15 mmol, or 1.7 g/day for an average man. The amount is remarkably constant and depends on the amount of muscle in the body and, to a lesser extent, on the amount of muscle in the diet. Muscle mass is typically a smaller fraction of a woman's total body weight than of a man's, and the excretion of creatinine by a woman is generally less than the excretion of creatinine by a man of equal weight. This fact must be kept in mind in assessing the creatinine excretion of a patient.

A constant fraction of the creatine phosphate in the body is broken down each day to form creatinine. This constancy is useful in testing the reliability of 24-hour urine samples and is widely used to assess the amount of skeletal muscle present. In addition, it is a useful denominator for other measurements of urinary metabolites. When muscles degenerate because of muscular dystrophy or paralysis, the creatinine content of the urine decreases because the body pool of creatine decreases.

The Excretion of Nitrogenous Wastes

Ammonia, as we have seen, is derived from glutamine in the kidney by the action of glutaminase. The amount of ammonia in the urine varies with the degree of acidosis in the patient. Urea is formed primarily from the amino groups of amino acids and is also formed from the nitrogens released in the breakdown of pyrimidines. The amount of urea in the urine is increased by a diet rich in protein. Urinary uric acid in the human, as we shall see, is derived from the breakdown of purines and is increased in those clinical conditions in which the turnover of nucleotides is increased, such as leukemia, polycythemia, sickle cell anemia, and cancer. Urinary creatinine, derived from creatine or phosphocreatine, reflects the muscle mass of the patient. The amount in the urine is initially increased when muscles are breaking down in muscular dystrophy. Then, as the muscle mass becomes decreased, the excretion of creatinine also decreases.

Synthesis of Porphyrins

The synthesis of heme proteins, such as hemoglobin, cytochromes, and catalase, involves not only the synthesis of the peptide chains of the protein components, but also the synthesis of the porphyrin ring. This is produced by the condensation of four molecules of the pyrrole, porphobilinogen, which in turn is synthesized from glycine and succinyl CoA. The first step in the biosynthesis of the pyrrole ring is the condensation of glycine and succinyl CoA to form α-amino-β-ketoadipic acid, which undergoes decarboxylation to form δ-aminolevulinate. This reaction, catalyzed by δ-aminolevulinate synthetase, is the committed step in the biosynthesis of porphyrins and an important control site. The decarboxylation step is catalyzed by an enzyme that is located in the endoplasmic reticulum and requires pyridoxal phosphate as cofactor.

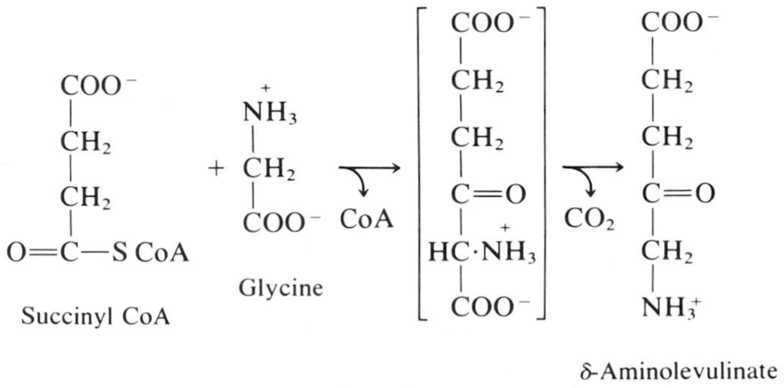

δ-Aminolevulinate

Two molecules of δ-aminolevulinate condense in a reaction catalyzed by porphobilinogen synthetase (also known as δ-aminolevulinate dehydratase) to form porphobilinogen. Two covalent bonds are formed and 2 mol water are removed.

Porphobilinogen

This enzyme-catalyzed reaction involves the intermediate formation of a Schiff base between the keto group of one molecule of δ-aminolevulinate and the ε-amino group of a lysine residue in the enzyme. Both the δ-aminolevulinate synthetase and the porphobilinogen synthetase are inhibited by heme, hemoglobin, and other heme proteins.

Four molecules of porphobilinogen condense head to tail to form a linear tetrapyrrole that remains bound to the enzyme uroporphyrinogen synthetase. An ammonium ion, NH_4^+, is released for each methylene bridge formed. The linear tetrapyrrole cyclizes and loses another ammonium ion as the ring is completed. The product is uroporphyrinogen III. The synthetase requires a second protein, an isomerase termed cosynthetase, in order to catalyze the synthesis of uroporphyrinogen III. This is the first of a series of modifications of porphyrin rings that result in the heme portion of hemoglobin. The side chains of uroporphyrinogen III are arranged asymmetrically. If only the synthetase is present, the symmetric isomer uroporphyrinogen I is produced; the isomerase carries out the isomerization of one of the pyrrole rings to yield the asymmetric uroporphyrinogen III. Several subsequent reactions, decarboxylations and oxidations, alter the side chains of the porphyrin skeleton and the degree of saturation of the porphyrin ring to yield protoporphyrin IX, the heme group of hemoglobin.

Protoporphyrin IX can react spontaneously with iron at a very low rate. A specific iron-inserting enzyme, ferrochetalase, catalyzes the addition of iron to yield protoheme IX, heme. This can react with oxygen to form protohemin IX, which inhibits the condensation of succinyl CoA and glycine to form δ-aminolevulinate. Thus protohemin IX is a feedback inhibitor of the entire reaction sequence. Normally, the protohemin combines with globin to form hemoglobin, and the concentration of free protohemin is less than that required for feedback inhibition. The enzyme heme synthetase assembles ferrous iron, protoporphyrin, and the globin protein to form hemoglobin.

INHERITED DISORDERS OF PORPHYRIN METABOLISM

There are several inherited disorders of porphyrin metabolism. In congenital erythropoietic porphyria, there is a deficiency of uroporphyrinogen III cosynthetase, the isomerase that yields the asymmetric isomer when the liner tetrapyrrole undergoes cyclization. To obtain the required amount of uroporphyrinogen III, large quantities of uroporphyrinogen I are formed, even though this symmetric isomer itself has no physiologic role. Uroporphyrin I, coproporphyrin I, and other symmetric derivatives accumulate. The disease, transmitted as an autosomal recessive trait, causes the patient to excrete urine that is red in color because of the large amounts of uroporphyrin present. In addition, the patient's teeth have a strong red fluorescence under ultraviolet light because of porphyrins deposited in the teeth. The spleen is enlarged, and the patient is sensitive to light.

A totally different disease, acute intermittent porphyria, involves a markedly elevated activity of δ-aminolevulinate synthetase in the liver. As a result, the concentrations of aminolevulinate and porphobilinogen in the liver are increased, and large amounts are excreted in the urine. Inherited as an autosomal dominant trait, this disease is characterized by intermittent abdominal pain and neurologic disturbances. An experimental model of this disease can be produced by injecting an animal with allylisopropyl acetamide, which causes a marked elevation of δ-aminolevulinate synthetase, an overproduction of porphyrins, and porphyria.

DEGRADATION OF HEME

The normal human erythrocyte has a life span of approximately 120 days. Old cells are removed from the circulation and degraded in the spleen. The protein part of hemoglobin is hydrolyzed to its constituent amino acids. Heme undergoes cleavage of its α-methene bridge to yield the linear tetrapyrrole biliverdin. This reaction is catalyzed by heme oxygenase, a mixed function oxidase that uses molecular oxygen and NADPH. It is a microsomal enzyme coupled to a cytochrome P_{450} electron transport chain very similar to that involved in the hydroxylation of steroids. The central methene bridge of biliverdin is reduced by biliverdin reductase to form bilirubin. The reductant is NADPH.

Bilirubin is transported to the liver in a complex with serum albumin. There it is made more soluble by condensation with glucuronic acid residues donated by uridine diphosphoglucuronate (UDPGA). Bilirubin accepts two glucuronate residues, forming bilirubin diglucuronide, which is excreted in the bile. The conjugation involves the joining of the carboxyl group of the propionic acid side chain of bilirubin with an OH group of the glucuronic acid.

In the Crigler–Najjar syndrome, a rare and recessively inherited syndrome, the liver lacks the enzyme that catalyzes this reaction, bilirubin UDP glucuronyl transferase. This results in jaundice, the accumulation of bile pigment in the plasma in an amount great enough to impart a yellowish tint to the skin and the whites of the eyes. Jaundice is not a disease itself, but a symptom of underlying disease.

When the liver is damaged, as in hepatitis or cirrhosis, the hepatic cells lose some of their ability to remove bilirubin from the circulation and to form the diglucuronide. The level of bilirubin in the plasma and tissues rises, and jaundice results.

The ability of the neonatal liver to conjugate bilirubin is limited, presumably because bilirubin UDP glucuronyl transferase is relatively inactive in the first few days of life. This results in a short-lived jaundice, which usually clears up spontaneously as the enzyme activity increases after birth. If there is a severe deficiency of the enzyme, however, the bilirubin may precipitate in the brain and cause permanent damage (kernicterus). Irradiating such infants with blue light, which activates and degrades bilirubin, has proved to be therapeutically effective. The capacity of the liver to conjugate bilirubin normally increases rapidly in the first few days of life, suggesting that bilirubin induces the synthesis of the transferase.

In the biosynthesis of heme, glycine contributes all the nitrogen atoms of the heme ring. The carboxyl carbon of glycine is lost as carbon dioxide in the formation of δ-aminolevulinate. The methylene carbons of the eight glycines involved in the synthesis of one porphyrin ring are incorporated into the ring structure. Four become the methylene bridge carbons and the other four become carbon 2 of each pyrrole ring, adjacent to the nitrogen atom. All the other carbon atoms are derived from succinyl CoA.

ONE-CARBON COMPOUNDS

Just as CoA is a carrier of activated two-carbon units, tetrahydrofolate is a carrier of activated one-carbon units. Tetrahydrofolate consists of a substituted pteridine ring linked by *p*-aminobenzoate to glutamate.

Pteridines were first discovered as pigments in butterfly wings and as eye pigments in the fruit fly, *Drosophila*. Humans are unable to synthesize the pteridine ring and obtain tetrahydrofolate from microorganisms in the gut. The one-carbon group is attached to tetrahydrofolate at its nitrogen-5 or nitrogen-10 position, or at both. It can be attached to tetrahydrofolate in any one of three oxidation states. The most reduced form is a methyl group; the intermediate stage of oxidation is a methylene group; and the most oxidized state is either a methenyl, formyl, or formimino group. A fourth one-carbon unit, the most oxidized of all, is carbon dioxide; in transfer reactions, this unit is bound to biotin rather than to tetrahydrofolic acid (THFA).

All these one-carbon units are interconvertible (Fig. 5–10). N^5, N^{10}-methylene tetrahydrofolate can be reduced to N^5-methyl tetrahydrofolate or oxidized to N^5, N^{10}-methenyl tetrahydrofolate. The latter can be converted to N^5-formimino tetrahydrofolate and to N^{10}-formyl tetrahydrofolate, which are at the same level of oxidation. N^{10}-formyl tetrahydrofolate can be synthesized from formate and ATP. These compounds donate one-carbon units in a variety of biosynthetic reactions, such as the synthesis of the purine ring.

Fig. 5–10. *Interconversions of the several kinds of tetrahydrofolic acids (THFA).*

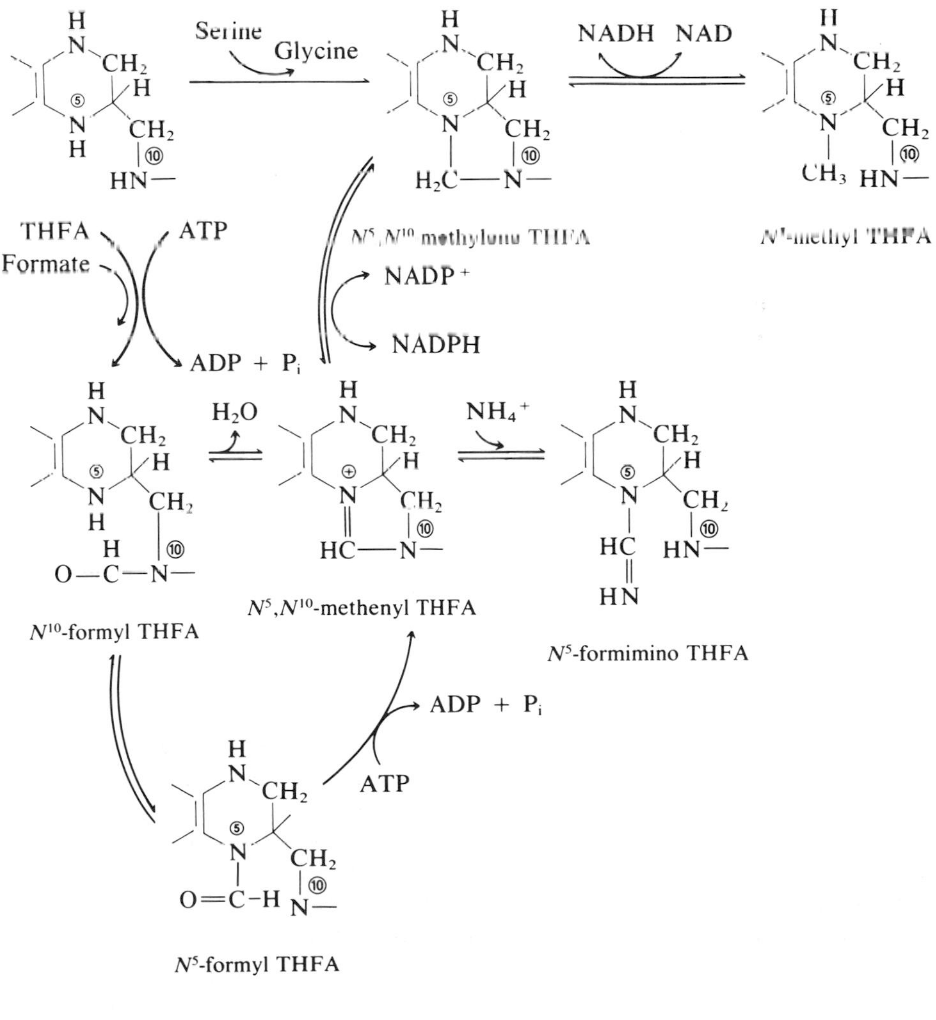

Although some one-carbon compounds at the methyl level of oxidation are bound to tetrahydrofolate, the major donor of activated methyl groups is S-adenosyl methionine, which is synthesized by the transfer of an adenosyl group from ATP to the sulfur atom of methionine.

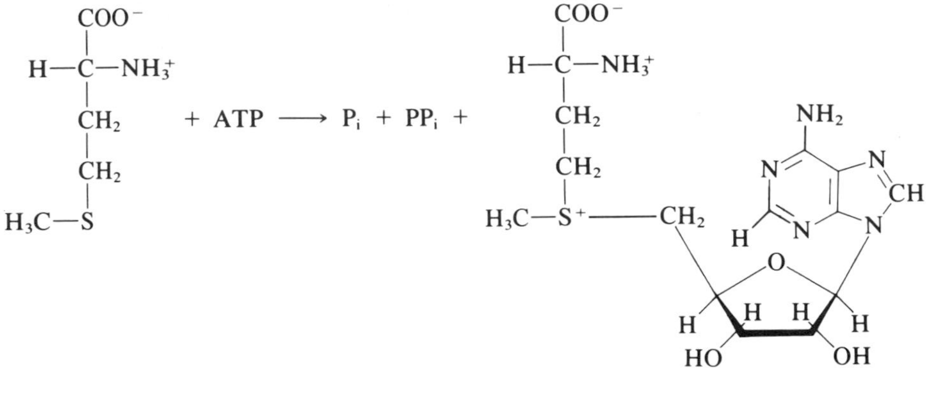

S-adenosyl methionine

The methyl group of the methionine unit in this sulfonium compound is activated and has a high enough transfer potential to be donated to other compounds. After it has donated its methyl group, S-adenosyl methionine becomes S-adenosyl homocysteine. This is hydrolyzed, and the homocysteine can accept the methyl group from N^5-methyl tetrahydrofolate and be reconverted to methionine. This accepts an adenosyl group from ATP, and S-adenosyl methionine is regenerated.

ASSEMBLY OF THE PURINE RING

The biosynthesis of the purine ring resembles the biosynthesis of cholesterol in that the molecule is put together piece by piece from a variety of precursors by a sequence of enzymatic reactions. Current understanding of these biosynthetic reactions came from experiments by John Buchanan, Robert Greenberg, and their colleagues. They fed various isotopically labeled precursors to birds and determined where the labeled atoms were incorporated into the purine ring. Birds were used because they excrete nitrogen largely in the form of uric acid, a purine derivative that is easily isolated in pure form. These experiments showed that glycine is the source of carbons 4 and 5, as well as nitrogen 7. Nitrogen 1 is derived from the amino group of aspartate; nitrogens 3 and 9 are derived from the amide group of the side chain of glutamine. Activated derivatives of tetrahydrofolate supply carbons 2 and 8, and carbon dioxide is the source of carbon 6.

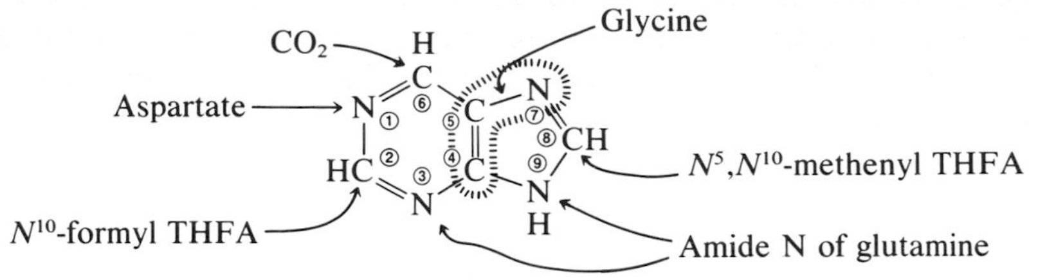

The ribose phosphate of both purine and pyrimidine nucleotides is derived from 5-phosphoribosyl-1-pyrophosphate (PRPP), which is synthesized from ribose-5-phosphate formed in the pentose phosphate pathway and from ATP. The pyrophosphate group is transferred from ATP to carbon 1 of ribose-5-phosphate, yielding PRPP.

The committed step in the synthesis of purine nucleotides is the formation of 5-phosphoribosyl amine from PRPP and the amide nitrogen of glutamine. The amino group from the side chain of glutamine displaces the pyrophosphate group attached to carbon 1 of PRPP with an inversion of the configuration so that the resulting carbon–nitrogen bond has the β-configuration. The reaction is driven by the hydrolysis of the pyrophosphate product.

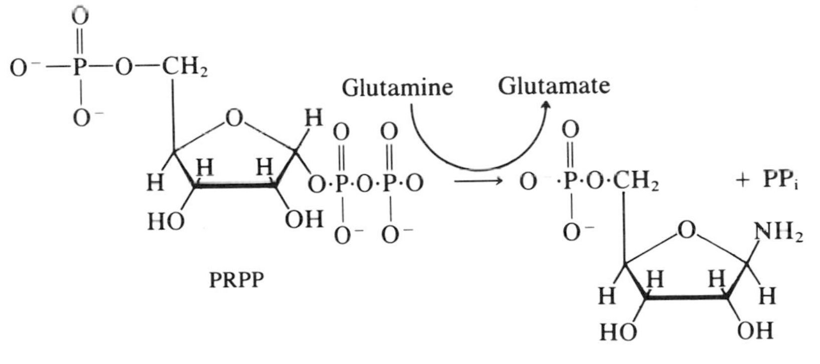

5-Phosphoribosyl amine

Glycine joins phosphoribosyl amine to yield glycineamide ribonucleotide. The reaction uses 1 mol ATP in forming the amide bond. The α-amino terminus of glycine reacts with N^5, N^{10}-methenyl tetrahydrofolate to yield α-N-formyl glycine amide ribonucleotide. The amide group is converted to an amidine group. The nitrogen, which becomes nitrogen 3 of the purine ring, is derived from the amide group of glutamine in a reaction that requires ATP. The product, formyl glycine amidine ribonucleotide, undergoes ring closure to yield 5-aminoimidazole ribonucleotide.

Glycine amide
ribonucleotide

Formyl glycine amidine
ribonucleotide

5-Aminoimidazole
ribonucleotide

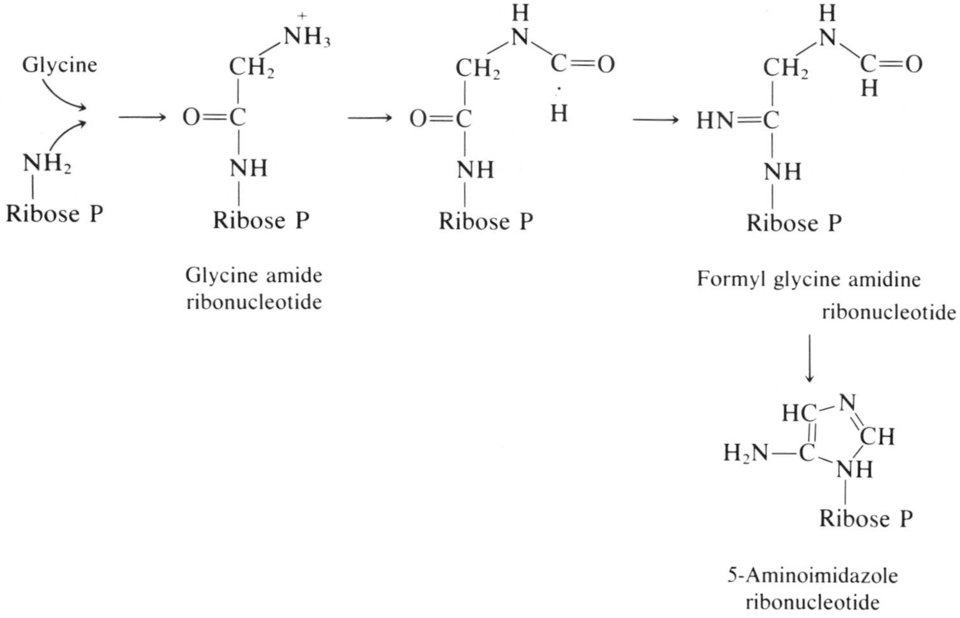

In the next step, a carbon atom from carbon dioxide carboxylates aminoimidazole ribonucleotide, forming 5-aminoimidazole-4-carboxylate ribonucleotide. This compound reacts with aspartate to form 5-aminoimidazole-4-N-succinocarboxamide ribonucleotide. This reaction is similar to the formation of arginosuccinate in the urea cycle; and ATP is required to drive it. The carbon skeleton of the aspartate is then split off as fumarate (as in urea synthesis) leaving the amino group behind as 5-aminoimidazole-4-carboxamide ribonucleotide. Aspartate contributes only its amino nitrogen to the purine ring.

In the final step, the carbon atom from N^{10}-formyl tetrahydrofolate is added to the amino group of the nitrogen that eventually becomes nitrogen 3 of the purine ring. This compound, 5-foramidoimidazole-4-carboxamide ribonucleotide, then undergoes dehydration and ring closure to form inosinate, which has the complete purine ring. The purine base of inosinate is called hypoxanthine.

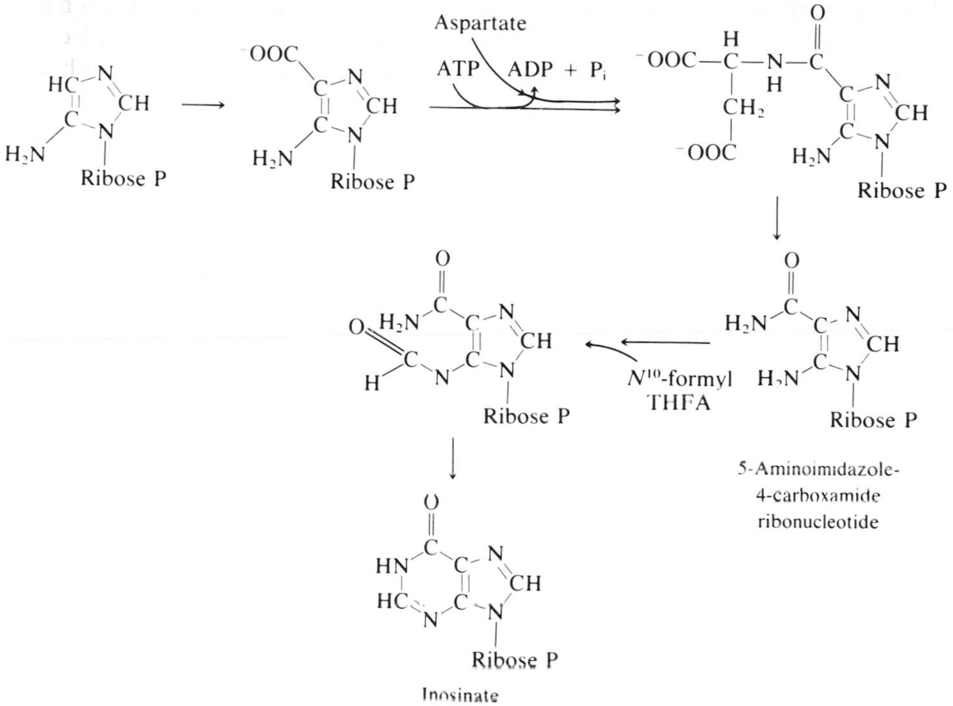

Inosinate

Inosinate is the precursor of adenylate (AMP) and of guanylate (GMP). Adenylate is synthesized from inosinate by the insertion of an amino group at carbon 6 in place of the carbonyl oxygen. The amino group is transferred from aspartate by the formation of an intermediate adenylosuccinate and the cleavage of fumarate from this compound.

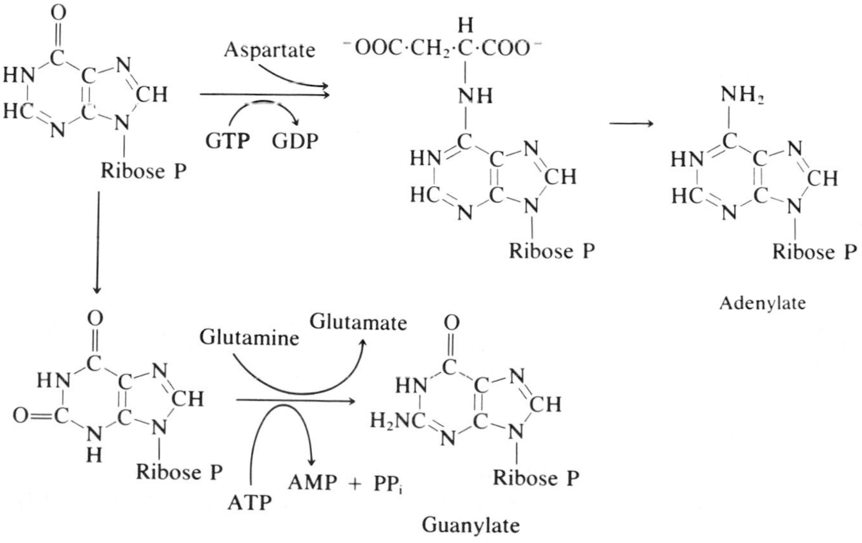

Guanylate, GMP, is synthesized by the oxidation of the hypoxanthine ring to xanthine with the insertion of an oxygen function at carbon 2. The oxygen is replaced by an amino group donated by glutamine. This reaction is driven by the cleavage of ATP to AMP and inorganic pyrophosphate, which is then hydrolyzed.

Regulation of Purine Formation

The production of inosinic acid is regulated at the early step in which an amino group is transferred from glutamine to PRPP. The enzyme glutamine PRPP amidotransferase is feedback-inhibited by many purine ribonucleotides. It appears that there are two regulatory sites: one binds ATP, ADP, or AMP, and the other binds GTP, GDP, or GMP. The inhibition is cumulative so that the presence of both types of purine nucleotides in high concentrations inhibits the enzyme more than the presence of either one alone in a high concentration. Thus all eventual products, the adenylates and the guanylates, inhibit the formation of purines by acting on the same site in the biosynthetic pathway, (i.e., the first committed step in the biosynthesis of inosinic acid).

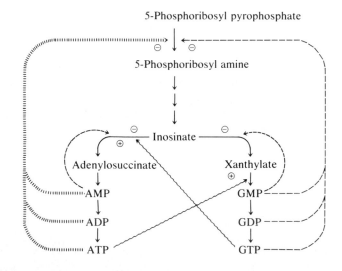

The branching pathways to AMP and GMP are regulated in a rather unusual fashion. The reaction pathway leading to guanylate requires ATP as a reactant, and that leading to adenylate requires GTP as a reactant. Thus an excess of ATP accelerates the synthesis of guanylate, and an excess of GTP accelerates the synthesis of adenylate. This reciprocal arrangement helps balance the production rates of AMP and GMP. The levels of AMP and GMP are further coordinated by feedback inhibitions. The conversion of inosinate to adenylosuccinate is inhibited by AMP, and the conversion of inosinate to xanthylic acid is inhibited by GMP. In this second type of feedback inhibition, AMP and GMP each inhibit their own biosynthesis.

Degradation of Purines

The nucleotides in a cell undergo continuous turnover. They are hydrolyzed to nucleosides by nucleotidases, and the phosphorolytic cleavage of nucleosides to the free base and ribose-1-phosphate or deoxyribose-1-phosphate is catalyzed by nucleoside phosphorylases. The ribose-1-phosphate can be converted by phosphoribomutase to ribose-5-phosphate and used in the synthesis of PRPP. Some of the bases themselves can be reused to form nucleotides by what are called salvage pathways.

Adenylate is deaminated to inosinate and then converted to the free base hypoxanthine. Xanthine oxidase, a flavoprotein that contains both nonheme iron and molybdenum, oxidizes hypoxanthine to xanthine and oxidizes xanthine to uric acid. The oxidant in both reactions is molecular oxygen which is reduced to a superoxide radical, O_2^-. The enzyme superoxide dismutase then converts the superoxide radical to hydrogen peroxide and molecular oxygen.

$$2\ O_2^- + 2\ H^+ \xrightarrow{\text{Dismutase}} H_2O_2 + O_2$$

The resulting hydrogen peroxide is decomposed by catalase to yield water and molecular oxygen. Xanthine is also an intermediate in the formation of uric acid from guanine, which undergoes deamination to form xanthine.

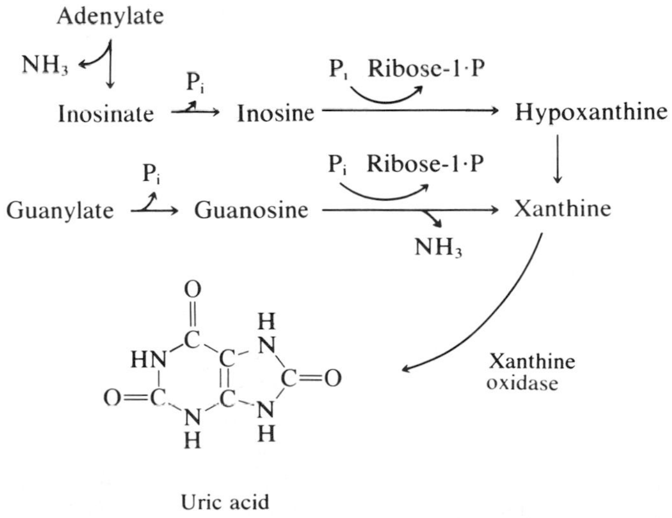

Uric acid

In humans, urate or uric acid is the final product of purine degradation and is excreted in the urine. Mammals other than primates have uricase, which cleaves uric acid to allantoin, a compound more water-soluble than urate. Lower vertebrates cleave allantoin to allantoic acid, while amphibians and some fish split allantoic acid to urea and glyoxylate. A progressive loss of enzymes has occurred in the evolution of primates and the loss of uricase has made us subject to attacks of gout, in which uric acid is deposited in cartilage, tendon, and joints. The urate is poorly water soluble and may precipitate out of urine forming kidney stones.

Salvage Pathways

The free purine bases adenine and guanine released by the hydrolytic degradation of nucleotides and nucleosides can be used in the synthesis of new purine nucleotides by salvage reactions that involve phosphoribosyl transferase. The ribose phosphate part of PRPP is transferred to the purine base to yield the corresponding nucleotide.

$$\text{Adenine} + \text{PRPP} \xrightarrow{\text{APRT}} \text{Adenylate} + \text{PP}_i$$

$$\text{Guanine} + \text{PRPP} \xrightarrow{\text{HGPRT}} \text{Guanylate} + \text{PP}_i$$

$$\text{Hypoxanthine} + \text{PRPP} \xrightarrow{\text{HGPRT}} \text{Inosinate} + \text{PP}_i$$

The salvage pathway requires much less energy than the reactions of the de novo synthesis of the purine ring. There are two salvage enzymes; adenine phosphoribosyl transferase (APRT), which specifically reacts with adenine and PRPP, and hypoxanthine guanine phosphoribosyl transferase (HGPRT), which reacts either with hypoxanthine or guanine to yield either inosinate or guanylate and pyrophosphate. The reaction is driven by the hydrolysis of the pyrophosphate.

Deficiencies of Purine Metabolism

KIDNEY STONES

When uric acid (urate) is cleared from the blood to be excreted in the urine, the amino groups that were added to the adenine and guanine rings are removed. Some are transferred the general nitrogen pool; some are excreted as ammonia or urea. Undissociated uric acid has a relatively low water solubility, about 0.1 g/liter water at 38°, and may precipitate in the urine, forming stones in the kidney or bladder. Kidney stones are usually calcium oxalate or calcium phosphate, but calcium urate may contribute to the formation of stones. The amount of urate excreted per day, about 2 to 4 mmol (0.3 to 0.6 g) is an index of purine turnover.

This is not an absolute estimate of total purine turnover, however, for part of the urate in the blood passes into the gut in gastric juice and bile. It is decomposed in the gut to ammonia, which may be reabsorbed and eventually excreted in the urine as urea.

GOUT

An increased concentration of uric acid in the tissues, because of either increased purine production or impaired purine excretion, may result in the deposition of crystals of urate in the tissue, especially in or near cartilages, tendons, and joints. For example, a small nodule of uric acid crystals, called a tophus, is common in the ear lobe. Gouty arthritis is marked by attacks in which the deposition of uric acid causes inflammation, swelling, and pain. Such attacks usually subside, and some of the uric acid may be reabsorbed.

At one time, gout was thought to be caused by overindulgence in rich foods and alcohol, but this is at most a contributory factor, not the primary cause. Gout is primarily a disease of adult males; less than 5% of gouty patients are women. The condition is at least in part hereditary, and the male relatives of gouty patients usually have elevated amounts of uric acid in the plasma. Normal levels of uric acid in plasma are approximately 4 mg/100 ml in women and 5 mg/100 ml in men. Most cases of gout arise from an overproduction of uric acid, although some patients have a partial deficiency of HGPRT, the enzyme that catalyzes the salvage pathway of nucleotide synthesis. The gene for HGPRT is located in the X chromosome, which may partly explain the higher frequency of gout in men. The deficiency of HGPRT and the resulting decreased synthesis of inosinic acid leads to an increased synthesis of PRPP, for PRPP synthetase is regulated by feedback inhibition by inosinic acid.

Gout is treated with allopurinol, probenecid (Benemid), and colchicine. Allopurinol is an analog of hypoxanthine and specifically inhibits xanthine oxidase, thereby decreasing the production of uric acid from xanthine and hypoxanthine. These are more soluble than uric acid and thus more readily excreted. Allopurinol may react with PRPP, forming allopurinol nucleotide, thus lowering the concentration of PRPP. Benemid is uricosuric, increasing the excretion of uric acid. Colchicine has been used in treating gout for many years, but its mechanism of action is unclear. It interferes with microtubules and inhibits leukocyte function, but the relationship of these actions to gout is unknown.

LESCH–NYHAN SYNDROME

A rare hereditary lack of the enzyme HGPRT results in the Lesch–Nyhan syndrome. It is inherited by an X-linked gene and affects only males. It is characterized by greatly elevated levels of uric acid in blood and urine, excessive production of uric acid, and certain striking neurologic features, including aggressive behavior, self-mutilation, mental retardation, and spasticity. Lesch–Nyhan patients bite off the tips of their fingers or bite their lips and may attack others. The compulsive self-destructive behavior of Lesch–Nyhan children appears at age 2 to 3 years. The tendency to self-mutilation may be so extreme that they must be protected by wrapping their hands in gauze or by splinting their arms so they cannot get their fingers into their mouths.

The reason that the deficiency of this enzyme, which is normally involved in the salvage pathway of purines, should lead to these bizarre behavioral changes is not at all clear. The missing enzyme normally salvages guanine and hypoxanthine and converts them to the corresponding nucleotides. HGPRT is especially active in the brain, whereas the other salvage enzyme, APRT, is only one-third as active in the brain as it is in the liver. This raises the possibility that guanine nucleotides have some special metabolic role in the nervous system that has not yet been recognized and that an individual deprived of the HGPRT salvage pathway cannot synthesize enough guanine nucleotides in the brain to maintain normal behavior. Lesch–Nyhan patients have elevated rates of de novo synthesis and turnover of purines and tend to be gouty. Allopurinol diminishes the synthesis of uric acid in Lesch–Nyhan patients, but it does not alleviate the neurologic features of the disease. The fact that such abnormal behavior can be caused by the absence of a single enzyme may have important implications for the future development of psychiatry.

PYRIMIDINE SYNTHESIS

In contrast to the de novo synthesis of purines, which begins with the attachment of ribose phosphate to nitrogen 9, the pyrimidine ring is completely assembled before it reacts with PRPP to form the nucleotide. The pyrimidine ring is formed by the condensation of carbamoyl phosphate and aspartate. The carbamoyl phosphate used in the synthesis of pyrimidines is produced in the cytosol, with glutamine as the nitrogen donor:

Glutamine $+$ 2 ATP $+$ HCO$_3^-$ $\rightarrow$

$\qquad$ Carbamoyl phosphate $+$ 2 ADP $+$ P$_i$ $+$ Glutamate

Carbamoyl phosphate condenses with aspartate in a reaction catalyzed by aspartate carbamoyl transferase, the committed step in the biosynthesis of pyrimidines.

$$
\underset{\text{Carbamoyl phosphate}}{H_2N-\overset{\overset{O}{\|}}{C}-O-\overset{\overset{O}{\|}}{\underset{\underset{O^-}{|}}{P}}-O^-} + \underset{\text{Aspartate}}{H_2N-\overset{\overset{H}{|}}{\underset{\underset{\underset{COO^-}{|}}{CH_2}}{C}}-COO^-} \longrightarrow \underset{N = \text{Carbamoyl aspartate}}{H_2N-\overset{\overset{O}{\|}}{C}-\overset{\overset{H}{|}}{\underset{\underset{H}{|}}{N}}-\overset{\overset{H}{|}}{\underset{\underset{\underset{COO^-}{|}}{CH_2}}{C}}-COO^-} + P_i
$$

The product, *N*-carbamoyl aspartate, undergoes cyclization with loss of water to yield dihydroorotic acid. This undergoes dehydrogenation with NAD as hydrogen acceptor to form orotic acid.

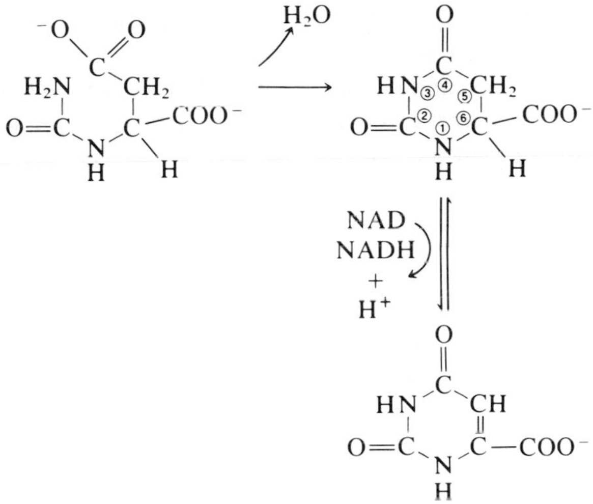

Orotic acid

Orotic acid then reacts with PRPP to form orotidylic acid. This reaction, catalyzed by orotidylate phosphorylase, is driven by the subsequent hydrolysis of pyrophosphate. Orotidylate undergoes decarboxylation to yield uridylic acid. CTP is formed from UTP by a reaction in which the carbonyl oxygen at carbon 4 is replaced by an amino group derived from glutamine. The reaction is driven by the conversion of ATP to ADP.

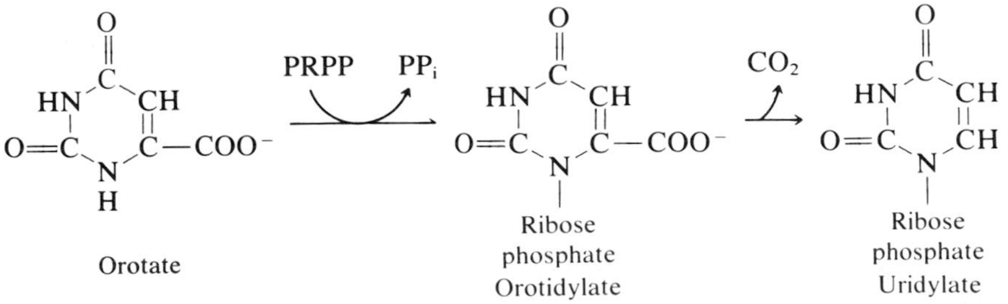

Orotate

Ribose
phosphate
Orotidylate

Ribose
phosphate
Uridylate

Control of Pyrimidine Nucleotide Biosynthesis

Aspartate carbamoyl transferase, which catalyzes the committed step in pyrimidine biosynthesis, is regulated by feedback inhibition by the product, UTP or CTP; the inhibition is prevented by ATP. The enzyme consists of catalytic subunits that bind the substrate and regulatory subunits that combine with the inhibitors UTP and CTP, as well as with ATP to prevent the inhibition. One further site of feedback inhibition is the enzyme PRPP synthetase, which catalyzes the synthesis of PRPP from ribose-5-phosphate and ATP. PRPP is a common precursor of both purine and pyrimidine nucleotides, and PRPP synthetase is inhibited by ADP, by GDP, and by pyrimidine nucleotides.

Orotic Acidemia

A hereditary deficiency of the enzymes orotidylate pyrophosphorylase or orotidylic decarboxylase, which convert orotic acid to uridine monophosphate, interferes with pyrimidine biosynthesis; orotic acid accumulates in blood and tissues, and excretion of the compound in the urine increases. A normal adult excretes orotic acid at a rate of 1.2 mg/24 hours; an individual with orotic acidemia excretes much more. The overproduction of orotic acid results from the lack of feedback inhibition by the product of the enzyme that catalyzes the committed step.

Orotic acidemia is characterized by retarded growth and development and by hypochromic anemia. Aspartate carbamoyl transferase is inhibited by CTP in *Escherichia coli* and by UTP in *Pseudomonas,* but the human enzyme is inhibited by uridine or cytidine. Thus the administration of uridine to a patient with orotic acidemia inhibits aspartate carbamoyl transferase and decreases the production of orotic acid. In addition, the uridine undergoes conversion to UTP and CTP.

Thymidylate Synthetase

DNA contains thymine (5-methyl uracil) rather than uracil. After uridylic acid has been reduced to deoxyuridylic acid, it is subsequently methylated to deoxythymidylate (dTMP) by the transfer of a one-carbon unit from N^5, N^{10}-methylene tetrahydrofolate, which also serves as an electron donor in this reaction. The product is not tetrahydrofolate but dihydrofolate; tetrahydrofolate is regenerated from dihydrofolate by a reaction catalyzed by dihydrofolate reductase:

$$\text{Dihydrofolate} + \text{NADPH} + \text{H}^+ \rightarrow \text{Tetrahydrofolate} + \text{NADP}^+$$

Certain analogs of dihydrofolate, such as aminopterin and amethopterin (methotrexate), are potent inhibitors of dihydrofolate reductase. These drugs are valuable tools in the treatment of certain forms of cancer, such as acute leukemia and choriocarcinoma. Rapidly growing cells require large amounts of thymidylate for the synthesis of DNA, and the conversion of deoxyuridylate (dUMP) to deoxythymidylate (dTMP) is blocked if tetrahydrofolate cannot be regenerated. Thus inhibiting the formation of thymidylate greatly retards the division of malignant cells.

Degradation of Pyrimidines

Pyrimidines undergo deamination and reduction of the double bond between carbons 5 and 6. The ring is opened between nitrogen 3 and carbon 4 to yield N-carbamoyl propionate (from cytosine or uracil) and N-carbamoyl isobutyrate (from thymine). These are converted to β-alanine and β-aminoisobutyrate, respectively, with the loss of NH_3 and carbon dioxide. Removal of the amino group yields carbon skeletons that eventually enter the tricarboxylic acid cycle. The nitrogens of pyrimidines are excreted in the urine as ammonia or urea (Table 5–1).

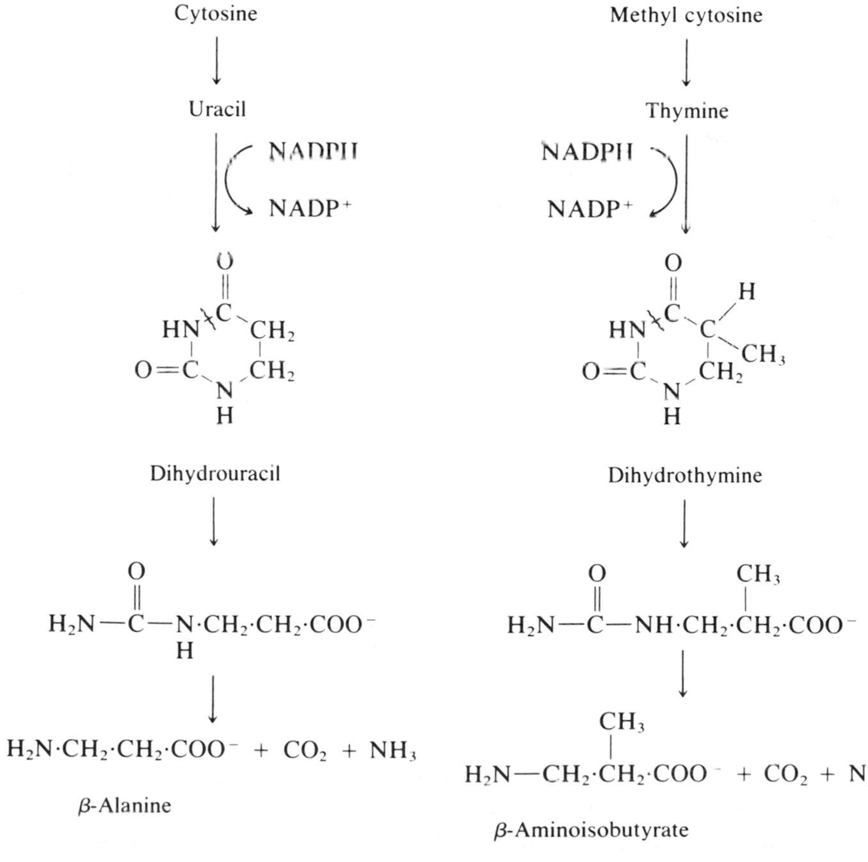

Table 5-1. *Metabolism of Purines and Pyrimidines*

	Purines	Pyrimidines
Precursors	Glutamine, Aspartate, Glycine, CO_2, Formyl THFA	Carbamoyl phosphate, Aspartate
PRPP added	As first step	After ring closure
First ring product	Inosinic acid	Orotic acid
Control	Feedback: AMP and GMP inhibit first step, transfer of amide group from glutamine to PRPP	Feedback: UTP inhibits Aspartate carbamoyl transferase
	Both purines and pyrimidines inhibit PRPP synthetase, ribose-5-P + ATP → PRPP + AMP	
Catabolism	Oxidation	Reduction with NADPH
Excretory product	Uric acid	Urea

POLYAMINES

Putrescine, Spermidine, and Spermine

The polyamines include a number of small organic cations that appear to play regulatory roles in the growth process. The major polyamines, putrescine, spermidine, and spermine, have long been known as components of putrifying matter and as components of seminal fluid. It is now recognized that these compounds are present in most, if not all, tissues and have an important role in stimulating the synthesis of RNA. In addition, the enzymes involved in the synthesis of the polyamines respond dramatically to hormonal stimulation. Thus, an important mechanism by which a hormone such as estradiol stimulates growth in its target tissues, such as the uterus or mammary gland, is by increasing the activity of the enzymes involved in the synthesis of polyamines. The polyamines stimulate RNA synthesis and therefore the growth process in these target tissues. In bacterial systems, as well as in mammalian systems, an increase in the biosynthesis of polyamines is one of the earliest events in cell proliferation.

Ornithine Decarboxylase

The conversion of ornithine to putrescine is catalyzed by ornithine decarboxylase, the rate-limiting enzyme in the biosynthesis of polyamines. This enzyme has one of the most rapid turnover rates of all mammalian enzymes, on the order of 15 minutes, and its messenger RNA has an equally brief half-time. The activity of this enzyme is increased by hormones that affect growth and is elevated in tumor cells, virus-infected cells, embryonic cells, and any other cell that is undergoing rapid growth. Spermidine and spermine are formed from putrescine and exert a feedback inhibition on ornithine decarboxylase.

In the synthesis of spermidine and spermine, S-adenosyl methionine is enzymatically decarboxylated to yield propylamine. This is added to putrescine by an aminopropyl transferase. A second mol of propylamine is added to the other end of spermidine to yield spermine. This reaction is catalyzed by an aminopropyl transferase different from that which catalyzes the synthesis of spermidine. The second aminopropyl group is also derived from S-adenosyl methionine by the action of S-adenosyl methionine decarboxylase. Both the polyamines themselves and the enzymes involved in their biosynthesis tend to be greatly elevated in all systems undergoing rapid growth.

6

Metabolic Interconversions and Controls

The pathways of glycolysis, the tricarboxylic acid cycle, fatty acid oxidation, and the urea cycle do not occur in a biochemical vacuum. In the cell, all or most of these sequences not only occur simultaneously, but also are interdependent in many ways. The products of the reactions of one sequence may serve as substrates for reactions in other sequences. Some reactions produce the energy that is needed to drive other reactions, and some produce protons, one-carbon compounds, acetyl groups, amino groups, or phosphate groups that are transferred to other compounds.

The rate of any metabolic reaction may be controlled by altering the amount of the enzyme that catalyzes it, that is, by regulating the rate of the enzyme's synthesis or by regulating the rate of its degradation. Both the rate of the enzyme's synthesis and its catalytic properties may be altered in response to specific hormones. A metabolic pathway may be controlled by altering the kinetic properties of the rate-limiting enzyme or control may depend upon the location of the enzyme within the cell.

BIOCHEMICAL HOMEOSTASIS

The human body has a variety of mechanisms to maintain specific constituents, such as glucose and calcium ion, at relatively constant levels in the blood and within the cell. The term *homeostasis* was coined to describe the physiologic reactions that, in response to some stress that tends to alter the constituents of the body, restore the normal concentration of materials in the fluid matrix of the body. Comparable regulatory devices provide for biochemical homeostasis within a cell.

The many constituents of the cell are in a dynamic state. A carbon atom that is part of a glucose molecule at one moment may subsequently become part of a fatty acid, a nucleotide, a steroid, or an amino acid. Nitrogen atoms are readily transferred from one substance to another, yet the concentration of each of these body constituents remains relatively constant. The molecular constituents of the cell are engaged in a gigantic square dance—they change partners, but the number of dancers remains relatively constant.

METABOLIC POOLS

Any given substance may be formed by more than one reaction and may be used by more than one reaction. All the molecules of a given substance within a cell are known as the "pool" of that substance. For example, there is a pool of glucose-6-phosphate, a pool of acetyl CoA, a pool of inorganic phosphate, and a pool of amino nitrogen. The concept of a pool implies that there is complete and rapid mixing of the constituents and that the molecules in the pool are equally available to all the reactions. This is difficult to demonstrate. In some instances, it has been possible to show that mixing is not complete and that there is more than one pool of a given substance within the cells. These pools may be partially mixed, but separated because they are located in different subcellular fractions, for example, in the mitochondria and in the endoplasmic reticulum.

The size of the metabolic pool of any compound can be estimated by measuring the dilution of an injected labeled substance. The glucose pool of normal and diabetic rats was estimated by administering labeled glucose intravenously and withdrawing successive blood samples. By measuring the dilution of the injected radioglucose by the nonlabeled glucose present in the body, it was possible to calculate that normal rats have approximately 130 mg glucose per 100 g body weight, whereas diabetic rats have approximately 250 mg glucose per 100 g body weight. By similar experiments in humans, it was possible to show that the pool of uric acid in a normal individual was approximately 1 g, whereas the pool of uric acid in a gouty patient was elevated three-fold or more. Such measurements become difficult to interpret, however, if the substance under consideration is rapidly used and converted to other materials.

FLUX OF MATERIALS THROUGH A METABOLIC PATHWAY

Our previous discussions of biochemical sequences have been primarily qualitative descriptions of a pathway. For a more complete picture of intermediary metabolism we should have some idea of the quantitative aspects of these metabolic pathways; that is, the flux of materials through the reaction sequence expressed perhaps as the number of moles metabolized per hour. The amount of material that can pass through a reaction sequence is determined by the rate (V_{max}) of the slowest enzyme in the multienzyme system and by the amount of that enzyme per cell. This, the so-called rate-limiting step, is the step at which the overall sequence can be controlled. The steady state in the biochemical sense is that in which there is a constant flux of materials through the system during the interval of an experiment. Obviously, one system may be in a steady state, while other systems are not. The closest approach to a steady state under experimental conditions is achieved by starved yeast cells or by freshly extracted ascites tumor cells.

METABOLIC INTERCONVERSIONS

A simplified overview of the interconversions of carbohydrates, fatty acids, and amino acids is given in Figure 6–1. With appropriately labeled substrates, it can be shown that some 60% of the glucose eaten by a rat or a human is converted to carbon dioxide and water. Some 30% is converted to lipids, and approximately 3% is converted to glycogen. The synthesis of fatty acids requires NADPH as hydrogen donor, and the prime source of NADPH is in the pentose phosphate pathway. If the body's ability to use glucose is impaired by starvation or by diabetes, the synthesis of lipids is impaired secondarily because of the decreased production of NADPH. Fat is deposited not only when the diet has a high lipid content, but also when it is rich in carbohydrates or proteins. Obesity results simply from overeating and not from eating any particular kind of diet.

Mammals cannot carry out the net synthesis of carbohydrates from fatty acids. Fatty acids are oxidized and converted to acetyl CoA, and this two-carbon compound must condense with oxaloacetate (four carbons) to form citrate (six carbons). As the carbons of the citrate progress around the tricarboxylic acid cycle, two molecules of carbon dioxide are released. The resulting oxaloacetate can be decarboxylated to yield phosphenol pyruvate (three carbons), which can be converted to glucose by gluconeogenesis. By these reactions, a labeled carbon atom originally present in a fatty acid can be incorporated into glucose or glycogen. There is no *net* synthesis of glucose from fatty acid, however, because the conversion of pyruvate to acetyl CoA and carbon dioxide is irreversible.

The pathway by which a compound is synthesized usually differs from the pathway by which it is degraded. For example, glucose and glycogen are synthesized and broken down by enzymatic sequences that differ in three key points. The synthesis and breakdown of fatty acids to two-carbon units also occur by different pathways that operate in different subcellular organelles. The synthesis and breakdown of polypeptide chains and of purine and pyrimidine rings occur by different sequences of enzymatic reactions. The existence of these different pathways for the synthesis and degradation of a substance allows the cell to control each one independently, an obvious advantage.

ENERGY INTERRELATIONS AND CONTROLS

One of the primary characteristics of all living organisms is their capacity to regulate their activities according to circumstances. This regulation can be achieved not only by the nervous and endocrine systems, but also by mechanisms that control metabolism at the level of the enzymes. Certain primitive forms of life have neither nerve cells nor hormones, but they clearly exhibit metabolic control. One enzyme may be controlled by its obligatory coupling with another enzyme. For example, the rate of oxidation may be controlled by its requirements for ATP. There is an

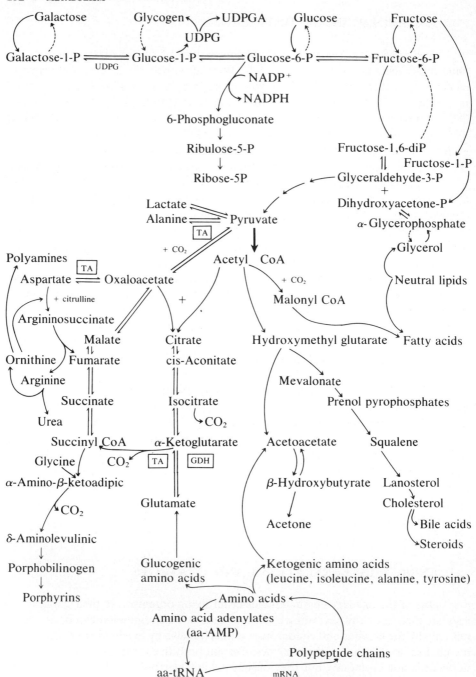

Fig. 6-1. *Metabolic interrelations.*

obligatory coupling between the transport of electrons from substrate to oxygen and oxidative phosphorylation; in other words, oxygen cannot be used unless inorganic phosphate and ADP are available. In turn, the supply of ADP and inorganic phosphate depends on the expenditure of energy through the cleavage of ATP.

Muscle expends energy and converts ATP to ADP and inorganic phosphate when it contracts. The concentrations of ADP and inorganic phosphate increase, and this increases the rates of glycolysis and of cellular respiration. When the muscle is not contracting, the transport of electrons is limited by the low concentration of ADP or inorganic phosphate required for this obligatory coupling. The control of cellular respiration by the concentration of ADP or inorganic phosphate can be readily demonstrated in isolated mitochondria. The rate of oxygen consumption by a mitochondrial system in vitro can be accelerated if hexokinase is added, because this enzyme catalyzes the conversion of ATP to ADP in the presence of glucose.

After the muscle has contracted and converted ATP to ADP and inorganic phosphate, oxidative phosphorylation is increased; in addition, the ADP and inorganic phosphate are reconverted to ATP. When essentially all the ADP is converted to ATP, the rate of oxidative phosphorylation falls to a low value.

When the contraction of muscle is stimulated under nervous control, muscle phosphorylase B, an inactive form, is converted to the active form, phosphorylase A. The phosphorylase A then catalyzes the breakdown of glycogen. The rate of glycogenolysis increases more than 1,000-fold when the rate associated with muscle in the tetanic state is compared with that associated with muscle at rest (Table 6–1). The rate of glycogenolysis in the tetanized muscle is of the same order of magnitude as the activity of phosphorylase in a muscle homogenate under optimal conditions of substrate concentration and pH. Even more amazing perhaps is the speed with which this enzymatic process returns to the resting state when the muscle relaxes.

FEEDBACK CONTROLS: NEGATIVE AND POSITIVE

The term *feedback control* is applied to the host of cellular mechanisms that regulate a reaction by using one of its products. The essence of negative feedback control is that some process, as it proceeds, brings about conditions that are

Table 6-1. *Glycogenolysis in Resting and Tetanic Frog Muscle*

	Decrease in Glycogen (mg/100 g muscle)	Rate (mg glycogen/ 100 g muscle/min)
Frog muscle at rest, 60 min	20	0.3
Frog muscle, 60 contractions in 6 min	68	11
Frog muscle, 60 contractions in 1 min	100	100
Frog muscle, 10 seconds tetanus	102	600

unfavorable for its continuation and, therefore, cause it to slow down or stop. In turn, the cessation of the process produces changes in the environment that tend to bring about the resumption of the process. Feedback controls may be either negative or positive, but most of the feedback controls in cells are negative.

Feedback controls prevent the overproduction of products and relate the rate at which a compound is synthesized to the rate at which it is used. For example, cytidylic acid inhibits the enzyme aspartyl transcarbamylase, which catalyzes the first step in the biosynthesis of cytidylic acid. This kind of feedback control helps explain the observation that externally supplied substrates may be preferentially incorporated into cellular constituents. In other words, the presence of a substance turns off the cellular biosynthetic mechanisms that normally produce it.

Another kind of control mechanism is product inhibition; the direct product of an enzyme reaction may inhibit the enzyme. For example, glucose-6-phosphate at concentrations as low as 5×10^{-4}M inhibits hexokinase. Thus, if there were an accumulation of glucose-6-phosphate within the cell for any reason, the activity of hexokinase would be decreased and less glucose-6-phosphate would be produced. Succinic dehydrogenase is inhibited not only by malonate, a dicarboxylic acid that competes with succinic acid for a site on the enzyme, but also by oxaloacetic acid. Oxaloacetate is bound to succinic dehydrogenase some 1,000 times more avidly than is the natural substrate, succinate. Even a small accumulation of oxaloacetate in the cell inhibits succinic dehydrogenase, decreases the rate of the tricarboxylic acid cycle, and depresses the production of oxaloacetate. The amount of oxaloacetate in the cell also regulates the use of acetyl CoA by condensing with it to form citrate.

CONTROL OF ENZYME RATES

The rate of any reaction depends on the number of active enzyme molecules present and on the rate at which each of these combines with substrate and releases the product. The rate at which enzyme molecules act may be influenced by

Temperature
Ionic strength
pH
Redox potential
Concentration of substrates, cofactors, and inhibitors
Concentration of specific cations, such as magnesium, calcium, and potassium

In the cells of higher organisms, temperature, pH, ionic strength, and most other physicochemical factors are relatively constant and are not of major importance in regulating enzyme rates.

The relation between the rate of an enzyme reaction and the concentration of its substrates is rather complex. The Michaelis–Menten equation (see Chapter

2) relates the velocity of the enzyme reaction and the concentration of substrate:

$$v = \frac{V_{max} \cdot [S]}{K_m + [S]}$$

In this equation, it is clear that the rate will be low and nearly proportional to substrate concentration when the concentration of substrate is low. The rate reaches half the maximal value V_{max} when the concentration of substrate equals K_m. The velocity approaches the maximal value V_{max} as the substrate concentration approaches infinity. At high concentrations of substrate, the rate of the reaction will be proportional to the amount of the enzyme. Both of these constants, V_{max} (the maximal velocity), and K_m (the substrate affinity), may be influenced by conditions such as pH and temperature. When assayed in vitro, each enzyme shows an optimal activity over a rather narrow range of pH.

CELLULAR COMPARTMENTATION

Each cell consists of a number of compartments that are more or less distinct biochemically as well as histologically. The channels in the endoplasmic reticulum are separated from the periluminal space, and the enzymes within the mitochondria are separated from those that lie outside the mitochondria. Certain enzymes appear to be distributed through all of the cell organelles, but most are restricted to one or a few of these compartments.

The enzyme that catalyzes a given reaction within the mitochondrion may have distinctly different properties from the enzyme that catalyzes a similar reaction in another part of the cell. If an enzyme within the mitochondrion uses a substrate produced in the nonparticulate fraction of the cell, the rate of the enzyme reaction may be limited by the rate at which the substrate can diffuse or be transported through the mitochondrial membrane. A number of shuttle mechanisms have evolved to transport specific substances, such as ATP or fatty acids, through the mitochondrial membrane.

COMPETITION BETWEEN ENZYMES FOR A COMMON SUBSTRATE

There are some key crossroad substances in intermediary metabolism, such as glucose-6-phosphate, pyruvate, acetyl CoA, and serine. Each of these may be converted into a number of other substances, each reaction catalyzed by specific enzymes. The direction that metabolism takes at these crossroad points depends on the relative amount of the substrate that combines with each of the specific enzymes. This is determined by the association constant between the enzyme and that substrate, by the relative amounts of the different enzymes, and by the turnover number of each enzyme. For example, the fraction of pyruvate that at any moment is converted to lactate, transaminated to alanine, carboxylated to oxaloacetate or malate, or decarboxylated to acetyl CoA depends on the relative amounts of each of the enzymes and the relative amounts of the specific cosubstrates or cofactors required for each of these reactions. The concentration of pyruvate becomes important when it is so low that not all the enzymes are fully saturated.

Suppose two enzymes use the same substrate and have the same maximal velocity, V_{max}, but the K_m of enzyme A is 10^{-4} M whereas the K_m of enzyme B is 10^{-3} M. When the substrate concentration is 10^{-5} M or less, the enzyme with a K_m of 10^{-4} M, enzyme A, will be reacting ten times as fast as the one with the K_m of 10^{-3} M, enzyme B. When the substrate concentration reaches 10^{-3} M the ratio of the two activities will be about 1.8 and, at 10^{-2} M, the two rates will be nearly equal.

The data in Table 6–2, obtained by Dickens and coworkers, concern the metabolism of glucose-6-phosphate in the liver. Since the K_m or the Michaelis–Menten constant of glucose-6-phosphate dehydrogenase is so much lower (1.3 × 10^{-5} M) than that for the isomerase (1.7 × 10^{-3} M), glucose-6-phosphate will be metabolized mostly by way of the pentose phosphate pathway at very low concentrations of glucose-6-phosphate. The V_{max} for glucose-6-phosphate dehydrogenase is low, 115 μmol/g liver per hour, so a relatively small but constant trickle of glucose units are metabolized this way. At higher concentrations of glucose-6-phosphate, it is metabolized by way of the isomerase (which has a high V_{max}, 7,600 μmol/g liver per hour) toward fructose-6-phosphate and by the mutase toward glucose-1-phosphate. Finally, at very high concentrations of glucose-6-phosphate, the enzyme glucose-6-phosphatase (K_m of 5 × 10^{-3} M) converts the excess glucose-6-phosphate back to glucose.

Enzymes may also compete with one another for a limited amount of a cofactor, such as NAD or NADPH. The concentrations of these cofactors may differ markedly in different parts of the cell. Clearly, an enzyme that requires such a cofactor and is located in that part of a cell with a high concentration of that cofactor has an advantage over an enzyme that requires the same cofactor but is located in a part of the cell where the concentration of the cofactor is lower.

Table 6-2. *Metabolism of Glucose-6-phosphate*

	V_{max} μmol G-6-P metabolized per g liver per hour)	Michaelis–Menten Constant (K_m)	ΔG (kcal/mol free energy change, pH 7)
Phosphoglucoisomerase	7,600	1.7 × 10^{-3} M	+0.5
Phosphoglucomutase	4,950	2 × 10^{-4} M	+1.7
Glucose-6-phosphate dehydrogenase	115	1.3 × 10^{-5} M	−5.5
6-Phosphogluconate dehydrogenase	124	1 × 10^{-5} M	−0.5
Glucose-6-phosphatase	1,100	5 × 10^{-3} M	−3.5

Enzyme sequences may be coordinated by coenzymes that are alternately oxidized and reduced. For example, one enzyme might catalyze the reaction:

$$AH_2 + NADP^+ \rightarrow A + NADPH + H^+$$

Another enzyme system might return the coenzyme to its oxidized state:

$$H^+ + NADPH + B \rightarrow BH_2 + NADP^+$$

There might be no other relation between substance A and substance B. For example, A might be glucose-6-phosphate, and B might be some intermediate in fatty acid synthesis that requires NADPH. Thus the rate at which fatty acids are synthesized is correlated with the rate of the pentose phosphate pathway; enzymatic control is achieved through a shared cofactor.

METABOLIC FATES OF THE β-CARBON OF SERINE

It is possible to describe which specific carbon atom of the precursor is incorporated into which specific position in the product molecule. For example, the β-carbon of serine has several possible fates (Fig. 6–2). Serine can be converted to 3-phosphoglycerate and then, by the reversal of glycolysis, can yield glucose labeled in carbon 1 and carbon 6. Serine can be converted to pyruvate, and the pyruvate undergoes oxidative decarboxylation to yield acetyl CoA. Then, in fatty acid synthesis, these acetyl CoA units are joined, and the β-carbon is incorporated into carbons 2, 4, 6, 8, 10, 12, 14, and 16 of palmitic acid—that is, in every other carbon atom. Serine can also be converted to glycerol, but its β-carbon becomes the terminal carbon of glycerol, called the α-carbon. Serine can undergo decarboxylation to ethanolamine, and this is converted to phosphatidyl ethanolamine. The β-carbon of serine then becomes the methoxy carbon of phosphatidyl ethanolamine and of phosphatidyl choline.

Serine can undergo a reaction to yield glycine plus the tetrahydrofolic acid derivative of its β carbon. Two moles of formyl tetrahydrofolic acid can be transferred to phosphatidyl ethanolamine to yield dimethyl phosphatidyl ethanolamine, which can then accept a third methyl group from S-adenosyl methionine to yield phosphatidyl choline. S-adenosyl methionine can be synthesized from 5,10-methylene tetrahydrofolic acid plus hydroxymethyl homocysteine. Thus, the carbon atoms of the entire molecule of phosphatidyl choline, its choline, glycerol, and fatty acid moieties, could be derived from serine. The β-carbon of serine can be converted by way of the formyl tetrahydrofolic acid derivative to carbons 2 and 8 of the purine ring and carbon 2 of the histidine ring.

In view of the alternative pathways available to the β-carbon, other than these direct ones, it is clear that the β-carbon could appear almost anywhere along the metabolic roadmap. When labeled serine is injected into a rat, the β-carbon of

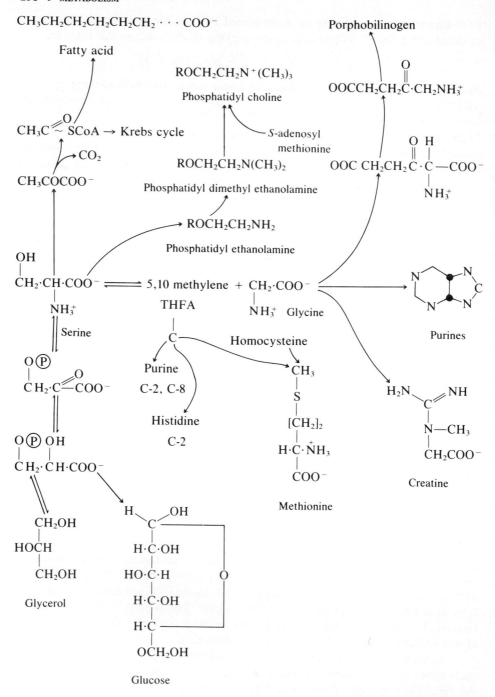

Fig. 6–2. *Metabolism of serine.*

serine appears in all the carbons of glucose, but it appears to the greatest extent in carbons 1 and 6. The other carbons have a much smaller amount of label derived by the action of the dicarboxylic acid shuttle and other metabolic byways.

Specific diseases may cause or may be caused by an interference in one or more of these metabolic pathways and their normal control mechanisms. An understanding of these pathways and of their control mechanisms is obviously of fundamental importance in the intelligent practice of medicine.

Bibliography

Devlin TM (ed): Textbook of Biochemistry with Clinical Correlations. New York, John Wiley, 1982
Text with clinical relevance.

Frisell WR: Human Biochemistry. New York, Macmillan, 1982
Text emphasizing human biochemistry.

Lehninger AL: Principles of Biochemistry. New York, Worth, 1982
A general review of biochemistry designed for first-time biochemistry students.

McGilvery RM: Biochemistry: A functional approach, 3 ed. Philadelphia, WB Saunders, 1983
Information on biochemistry with discussions on the relevance of biochemistry to the practice of medicine.

Newsholme EA, Leech AR: Biochemistry for the Medical Sciences. New York, John Wiley, 1984
Additional information on biochemistry emphasizing intermediary metabolism and its controls.

Smith EL, Hill RL, Lehman IR, et al: Principles of Biochemistry, 7 ed. New York, McGraw-Hill, 1983
A resource for standard biochemistry.

Stryer L: Biochemistry, 2 ed. San Francisco, WH Freeman, 1981
A clear and simple treatment of biochemistry.

Stanbury JB, Wyngaarden JB, Fredrickson DS, et al (eds): The Metabolic Basis of Inherited Diseases, 5 ed. New York, McGraw-Hill, 1983
Summaries of fundamental biochemistry underlying individual diseases, with detailed descriptions of cases.

Watson JD: Molecular Biology of the Gene, 3 ed. Menlo Park, California, Benjamin–Cummings, 1976
Fundamentals of biochemical genetics.

Index

Abortion, prostaglandins in, 96
Acetoacetate, free, 65–66
Acetone, 65–66
Acetyl CoA
  biologic oxidation and reduction, 37–38
  fatty acid synthesis and oxidation, 66–67
  from fatty acids, 65
  gluconeogenesis, 58
  oxidation of glucose, 35–37
  pyruvate conversion to, 42–43
  tricarboxylic acid cycle, 44–48
Acetyl group shuttle, mitochondrial membrane, 66
Acetyl phosphate, phosphate group transfer potential, 10
Acidosis, 105
Aconitase, 45
Actinomycin D, inhibition of estradiol effect, 89
Acute intermittent porphyria, 129
Acyl carrier protein, in fatty acid synthesis, 67
Adenine phosphoribosyl transferase (APRT), purine salvage, 138
Adenosine triphosphate, see ATP
S-Adenosyl methionine, 109, 132, 145, 157
Adenylate, 135–137
Adipocytes, 65
Adipose tissue, triacylglycerol storage, 66, 67
ADP
  passage across mitochondrial membrane, 53
  in respiratory control, 54

Adrenal cortex, hormonal maintenance, 84–86
Adrenocorticotropic hormone (ACTH), 84, 85
Adrenodoxin, 79, 84
Albinism, 121
Aldolase, 61
Aldosterone, 79, 82
  metabolism, 85
Alkaptonuria, 124–125
Amino acid oxidases, 102
Amino acids
  activation, 39
  branched chain, 112–116
  cofactors in reactions, 101
  deamintion, 102
  essential, 101–103
  fates within the cell, 100–101
  heterocyclic, 116–120
  interconversions, 151, 152
  specific transport systems, 100
  transamination, 102
  transport, Hartnup's disease, 117
  tricarboxylic acid cycle, 44
  uptake, 99–101
Aminotransferases, 102
Ammonia, 102, 127
  hyperammonemia, 109
  kidney, 105
  metabolism, 103–109
  toxicity, 105–106
AMP, branching pathways, regulation, 136
Androgens, 78, 85
  to estrogens, 83
Androstenedione, 82
  in virilization, 85